RT51 .N68 2009
0134111869894
Nightingale, Florence,

Notes on nursing : a
 guide for today's
     2009.

2009 09 01

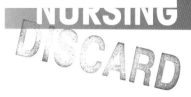

250101

D1059731

The International Council of Nurses has a long history, a worldwide membership, and an increasing number of diverse activities. But from its foundation in 1899 to the present day, its first objective has remained simple and unchanged. Briefly, this is to help in maintaining the highest standards of nursing in those countries which are in membership, and in helping those countries not yet in membership to improve their nursing care by education, legislation, and through professional organization.

International Council of Nurses

Commissioning Editor: Mairi McCubbin
Development Editor: Sheila Black
Project Manager: Susan Stuart
Designer: Kirsteen Wright
Illustration Manager: Bruce Hogarth
Illustrator: Jonathan Haste

$26.55

Notes on NURSING

A Guide for Today's Caregivers

International Council of Nurses
Geneva, Switzerland

Foreword by
The International Alliance of Patients'
Organizations (IAPO)

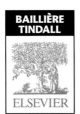

Edinburgh   London   New York   Oxford
Philadelphia   St Louis   Sydney   Toronto   2009

BAILLIÈRE
TINDALL
ELSEVIER

© International Council of Nurses 2009
© Illustrations Elsevier Limited 2009. All rights reserved.

No part of this publication may be reproduced or transmitted in
any form or by any means, electronic or mechanical, including
photocopying, recording, or any information storage and retrieval
system, without permission in writing from the Publisher.

Permissions may be sought directly from Elsevier's Rights Department:
phone: (+1) 215 239 3804 (US) or (+44) 1865 843830 (UK);
fax: (+44) 1865 853333; e-mail: healthpermissions@elsevier.com.
You may also complete your request online via the Elsevier website at
http://www.elsevier.com/permissions.

ISBN 978-0-7020-3423-7

British Library Cataloguing in Publication Data
A catalogue record for this book is available from the British Library

Library of Congress Cataloging in Publication Data
A catalog record for this book is available from the Library of Congress

Notice
Neither the Publisher nor the Author assumes any responsibility for
any loss or injury and/or damage to persons or property arising out
of or related to any use of the material contained in this book. It is
the responsibility of the treating practitioner, relying on independent
expertise and knowledge of the patient, to determine the best
treatment and method of application for the patient.

The Publisher

your source for books,
journals and multimedia
in the health sciences
www.elsevierhealth.com

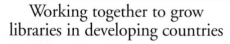

Working together to grow
libraries in developing countries

www.elsevier.com | www.bookaid.org | www.sabre.org

ELSEVIER   BOOK AID International   Sabre Foundation

The
publisher's
policy is to use
**paper manufactured
from sustainable forests**

Printed in Spain

Contents ...

Foreword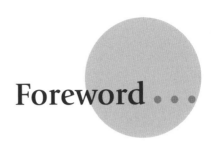

The International Alliance of Patients' Organizations (IAPO) is pleased to provide this Foreword to *Notes on Nursing*, the International Council of Nurses' guide for today's caregivers, and to reinforce the essential partnership between patients and caregivers. Caregivers provide a personal approach to healthcare, integral to a patient-centered system. This publication provides useful information on managing patients' daily needs and guidance for supporting patients in participating in their own care.

IAPO's Declaration on Patient-Centred Healthcare (2006)[1] outlines five principles of patient-centered healthcare which are relevant to the role of carers. These are respect, choice and empowerment, patient involvement in health policy, access and support, and patient information. In order to achieve patient-centered healthcare for patients with chronic conditions, these principles and the relationships between caregivers and patients are of paramount importance.

Chronic conditions often continue for many years and affect all aspects of a person's life. The goal for patients is to manage their condition so that they can participate in life as fully as possible. Caregivers play an important role by understanding patients' emotions, wishes and needs, and helping communicate these to others.

The updated *Notes on Nursing* supports effective dialogue between patients and caregivers to promote mutual understanding and respect, each contributing to achieve a good quality of life as defined by the patient.

Joanna Groves
Chief Executive Officer
International Alliance of Patients' Organizations (IAPO)

[1]Available online at www.patientsorganizations.org/declaration

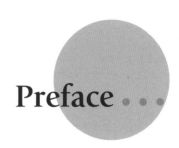

Preface

Florence Nightingale prepared her *Notes on Nursing* (see Figure 1.1) specifically for use by caregivers in the home. She knew that the lessons she had applied in nursing would also help equip providers of care in the home with methods and guidance to enhance the health of their patients. It was the women in families who were the main providers of care in her time, and so it was primarily to them that she offered this guidance.

Much has changed for caregivers and those they care for since that time. It is remarkable, however, how much of the advice in *Notes on Nursing* remains relevant. The approach to caregiving contained in the original *Notes* is timeless, even though the science and practice of healthcare have greatly evolved since its initial publication. It is for this reason that the International Council of Nurses and the Florence Nightingale International Foundation (FNIF) have prepared this modern edition of the *Notes* on the occasion of the 75th anniversary of the creation of the FNIF and 150 years after its original publication.

The intention has been to retain segments of the original work by Florence Nightingale that remain particularly relevant for caregivers today, while adding new information based on current medical knowledge and practice. In doing this, the ICN has been conscious that, although caregivers around the world are characterized first of all by the love and devotion they feel for those in their care, the reality is that they may work under conditions that are vastly different.

Some situations do not change, or only change slowly. The disparities in access to medications, professional services and expertise can be very different from one country to another, or even within regions of the same country. Many caregivers today will often be working under conditions that resemble those of their predecessors in Florence Nightingale's time, in terms of access to clean water, sewage treatment and lighting, as well as the layout of houses and rooms, and access to health professionals. Those fortunate enough to enjoy the 'modern' amenities of life will find that some of the advice in *Notes* does not suit their circumstances. Their counterparts in less fortunate material circumstances will, however, benefit from their utter applicability to maintaining health and well-being in the world as they know it. In both cases, the advice provided for caregiving based on compassion and empathy, still constitutes a valuable source of personal support and comfort for caregivers in fulfilling their demanding role.

The role of the caregiver remains an essential element of every country's system of care; all societies rely on the ability and willingness of individuals to provide personal care for those they love. In the industrialized economies this need is growing as increasing proportions of the population become old. It is estimated that, by 2050, more than 25% of the population in rich countries will be over 65 years old, compared to about 15% today. This aging of the population will also be felt in emerging economies. It is estimated that the percentage of the population of India and China that is over 65 years old will also have risen dramatically by 2050. Although public and private health-care services have an important role in ensuring the quality of their lives, many of the elderly in all societies will continue to depend upon family members and friends for care.

Other tragic realities underline the continuing importance of caregivers in our societies. For many patients suffering from AIDS and other diseases in developing countries, hospital care is not always affordable or accessible, and home-based public and private care services rarely exist. Therefore, most often the care for these patients falls on family members, especially on women. A United Nations report on Southern Africa revealed that two-thirds of caregivers in the households surveyed were female, and almost a quarter of them were over 60 years old. Home-based care is, by necessity, a strategy.

The advances in healthcare science and practice that have occurred since *Notes on Nursing* was written are not always available in every circumstance. There are many countries where knowledge of disease and how to deal with it exists, but where sanitary conditions, and access to health professionals and medication are often inadequate. It is with this unfortunate truth in mind that the modern edition of *Notes on Nursing* includes advice that Florence Nightingale offered at a time when living conditions in Europe were more difficult than they are now. Much of what she had to offer about sources of water, bedding, drainage, cleanliness and proper nutrition remains relevant for caregivers in many rural and remote parts of the world.

For the modern edition, ICN has gathered, from a variety of sources, additional information and advice based on developments in healthcare practice. We have included, for example, a section on the nature and treatment of infections. The original *Notes* was written before medical researchers confirmed the link between 'germs' and disease. There is advice for caregivers on the use and management of medications, which is necessary in view of the proliferation of the pharmacopeia available to modern medicine.

It is hoped that this modern edition complements the work of Florence Nightingale, extending the reach of her words to new generations of individuals committed to providing care that comforts and relieves the people whom they love.

Hiroko Minami
President of the International Council of Nurses (ICN)
Geneva, 2009

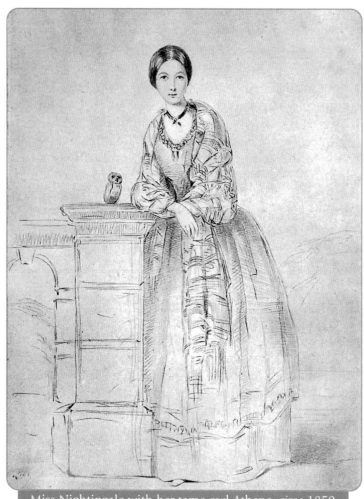

Miss Nightingale with her tame owl Athena, *circa* 1850, after a drawing by Parthenope Lady Verney

Courtesy of the Florence Nightingale Museum Trust

The Background to Florence Nightingale's *Notes on Nursing*

The original *Notes on Nursing* by Florence Nightingale was published in 1859, when she was nearly 40 and already a legend for her work to advance nursing and healthcare. In a letter to a friend she wrote about the book that: 'There is not one word in it written for the sake of writing but only forced out of me by much experience in human suffering.'

Her mission to care for wounded soldiers in the Crimean War had exposed her to the suffering generated by appalling standards of healthcare in military hospitals. Earlier work in British and French hospitals had revealed equally 'unhealthy' conditions. Her keen sense of observation, along with a talent for gathering facts and figures about what she observed, enabled her to draw conclusions that were prescient for her time.

The Crimean War experience confirmed her conviction about the link between good hygiene and illness. It did not take long for her to see that wounded soldiers who might recover were being killed by having to live in filthy conditions. She earned an almost saintly reputation for her work tending those wounded and dying soldiers. Queen Victoria wrote her letters of praise, and governments sought her advice. But it was the lessons she had learned about how to create environments that favored recovery and well-being that she valued and continued to apply later in

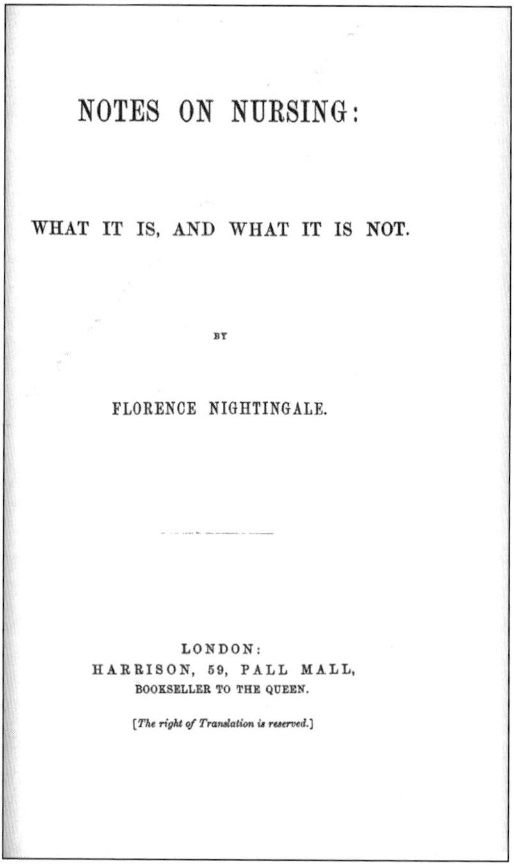

NOTES ON NURSING:

WHAT IT IS, AND WHAT IT IS NOT.

BY

FLORENCE NIGHTINGALE.

LONDON:
HARRISON, 59, PALL MALL,
BOOKSELLER TO THE QUEEN.

[*The right of Translation is reserved.*]

Figure 1.1
Title page of the original 1859 edition of *Notes on Nursing*

proposing reforms to how hospitals were built and how they should be managed.

The 'lady of the lamp'

Now the 'lady of the lamp' was offering in her *Notes* to caregivers some down to earth advice that ran counter to common beliefs and assumptions about illness, personal hygiene and healthy households. This small book caused

a sens
15,00
many
transl

Th
pour
pract
inna
patie
prac
reas
hea
on

firs
in
of

lessons she would later dispense, a
the basis of what knowledge she wa
nursing and caregiving could be

The vocation of Fl

Florence Nightingale
1820, in a villa rep
sojourn in Euro
them had ea
and fightin
Member
camp
be

model stressed causes
with some variants even invoking magic, diabolism, or lack
of discipline and moral control.

The miasma model centered on beliefs which considered
that illness was caused by poor hygiene and its consequences:
bad air and odors, rotting food, sewage, and lack of light
and fresh air. Under this model, treatment involved personal
and environmental cleanliness, access to fresh air, scrubbing,
boiling and bleaching. It was from this model of healthcare that Florence Nightingale began her work, applying
her talent for organization and an incisive mind to set out
a series of practices that were precursors of the future, when
research would at last reveal that a series of tiny microorganisms were in fact the agents of disease. The methods
of care that she devised before this was clearly understood
and accepted proved perfectly compatible with this discovery,
and remained an effective approach to combating 'germs,'
the enemies of good health and well-being. It is instructive
in reading her advice to caregivers to obtain a better grasp
of 'where she was coming from,' how she learned the

...d to understand on
...s able to determine how
...immeasurably improved.

...orence Nightingale

...was born in Florence, Italy, on 12 May
...ted by her British parents during a long
...pe. Her family was prosperous, and some of
...ned reputations for humanitarian principles
...g for lost causes. One grandfather was a British
...of Parliament for 46 years, during which time he
...aigned for the abolition of slavery and in favor of
...er conditions for sweathouse workers. She was brought
up and educated to be a proper British lady, groomed for
marriage and a conventional life in British high society. It
was a fate that troubled her, as she wrote in what she
called 'private notes,' which would become a life-long
habit. In one of these she confided that she felt herself
called to the service of humanity, and by 1840 she had
determined that this calling was to work in hospitals
among the sick. The very thought of such a vocation
appalled her family. Neither hospitals nor nursing were
respectable institutions at the time. She described hospital
conditions as she saw them in 1845:

*The floors were made of ordinary wood which, owing
to lack of cleaning and lack of sanitary conveniences
for the patients' use, had become saturated with
organic matter, which when washed give off the smell
of something quite other than soap and water. Walls
and ceilings were of common plaster also ... saturated
with impurity. Heating was supplied by a single fire at
the end of each ward, and in winter windows were kept
closed for warmth, sometimes for months at a time. In
some hospitals, half the windows were boarded up in
winter. After a time the smell became "sickening", walls*

streamed with moisture, and "a minute vegetation appeared". The remedy for this was "frequent lime washing with scraping", but the workmen engaged on the task "frequently became seriously ill".

In a letter Florence wrote in 1854, she describes the working conditions of nurses in these dreaded hospitals:

The Nurses … slept in wooden cages on the landing places outside the doors of the wards, where it was impossible for any woman of character to sleep, where it was impossible for the night nurse taking her rest in the day to sleep at all owing to the noise, where there was not light or air.

At the end of long days working in these impossible conditions, where some beds were known to be fatal to any patient assigned to them, she studied hospital reports, filling many notebooks with her conclusions on how this misery was propagated and how it could be fought. It was in the process of learning how to nurse, at a time when nursing schools did not exist, that she also made herself into one of the first experts in Europe on public hygiene and sanitary conditions.

By the age of 34 she was an experienced nurse, with skills and knowledge far in advance of the standards of the time. She was not married, which worried her family, although she had refused numbers of eager young men. A flattering portrait of her was painted in words by a friend, who described her as tall, very slight, with a willowy figure, thick brown hair, worn short, delicate coloring, gray, pensive eyes, perfect teeth. He said she had a sweet smile.

The war in the Crimea, which pitted the Russian Empire against Great Britain, France and the Ottoman Empire, created the crisis where her skills could be applied. Thousands of wounded soldiers were dying in filthy, makeshift hospitals for lack of treatment, lack of physicians and lack of food.

The newspaper reports from the front about these conditions provoked a public scandal in Britain. Florence obtained a commission from the government to lead a group of young women to the Crimea to care for the wounded.

The 40 nurses in her party arrived in the Crimea in 1854. What they found when they entered the dark rooms of the Barrack Hospital was revolting: young men, with often hideous wounds, lay in rows on unwashed floors crawling with vermin. There were no pillows, no blankets and no clean dressings for the wounds. Florence noted that, for the 1,000 men suffering acute diarrhea, there were only 20 chamber pots. One of her first tasks was to purchase 200 scrubbing brushes for washing the floors, which she and the other nurses did themselves at first, along with washing the sick men's clothes. Florence was adept at prying blankets, medications and food from wherever they could be found: 'I am a kind of General Dealer' she wrote.

By January 1855, after a number of calamitous battles, the number of wounded in the hospital had risen to 12,000 men. In letters they wrote home, her colleagues and the soldiers she treated described her as working herself to death, never sitting down for meals, working 20 hours at a time, dressing wounds and tending to the dying. Some days she spent 8 hours on her knees dressing wounds. It was her rule never to let any man who came under her observation die alone. That winter she attended to 2,000 such deaths.

'Nursing is the least of the functions into which I have been forced,' she wrote. The soldiers adored her; the physicians were dependent upon her. One of her nurses described accompanying her on a walk through the wards:

> As we slowly passed along the silence was profound;
> very seldom did a moan or cry from those deeply
> suffering fall on our ears. A dim light burned here and
> there, Miss Nightingale carried her lantern which she

would set down before she bent over any of the patients.
I much admired her manner to the men – it was so
tender and kind.

It was said that, for her sake, the troops gave up
swearing. It was work that could have crushed any other
person, but still she found energy for the administrative
work for which she was gifted and which no one else was
available to take on. In whatever time was left, she wrote
letters home for the soldiers. Inevitably, she collapsed,
hovering for 2 weeks between life and death. Admirers
around the world, who had followed accounts of her
devotion, prayed for her recovery. She had achieved much
in a short time, especially the one goal she held uppermost
from the moment she decided to go to the Crimea – to
transform the image of nursing by impressing upon it the
stamp of her own professionalism and dedication.
Nonetheless, she emerged from the war with a deep sense
of failure, because there was so much work left to be done.
She set herself to the tasks of creating a professional
nursing school, while also working to transform the world
of hospitals, military and public.

A systematic approach to providing care

Florence Nightingale's approach was always systematic and
empirical. What others only observed, she measured, counted,
collated and synthesized into trenchant conclusions,
combined with recommendations for action. Her personal
life was approached with the same clinical method. She
wrote at one point that it is necessary to decide for oneself:
what grievances one will bear as being unavoidable, what
grievances one will escape from, what grievances one will
try to remove.

From the volumes of her personal 'Notes' she assembled a
report for the government and the public on the reform of
hospitals. It began with the statement: 'It may seem a strange
principle to enunciate as the very first requirement in a

hospital that it should do the sick no harm.' She marshaled facts and figures to convince that the high mortality rates in hospitals were unnecessary and preventable. But her principal concern remained to establish nursing as a respected and respectable profession. It was during her campaign to establish a Training School for Nurses that she wrote *Notes on Nursing*, in her spare time. The slim volume caused a sensation, but the credibility of the source made it an instant success with caregivers everywhere, and it was translated into many languages. The indomitable spirit of Florence Nightingale infused her words with compassion, as she pleaded with caregivers to remember that the sick suffer almost as much mental as bodily pain. For the rest of her life, although made increasingly reclusive by illness, she advanced the cause of nursing, and the improvement of hospitals and public hygiene.

Her work inspired reformers everywhere. Henry Dunant, founder of the Red Cross and one of the originators of the Geneva Convention, spoke for many of his generation when he said that what had inspired him to dare such action was the example of Florence Nightingale in the Crimea. She died on 13 August 1910 at the age of 90 years and 3 months. In deference to her wishes for a simple burial, expressed in her will, the offer by the British government of a national funeral and burial at Westminster Abbey was declined.

Changes in the understanding of disease

Florence Nightingale's insights into the causes of disease and its propagation, and therefore the importance of fresh air, light, cleanliness and nutrition, were unusual when we consider the state of the medical arts when she wrote *Notes on Nursing* in the late 1850s.

Bacteria and other microorganisms had been observed by researchers in the late 17th century, but their link to illness was not appreciated. Although a method had been developed in 1796 to protect people from smallpox by exposing them to cowpox virus, no one knew why it worked. A French researcher, Louis Pasteur, suggested in a paper published in 1859 that microorganisms might be the cause of many human and animal diseases. This was a revolutionary idea. His work and that of other researchers led them to formulate the germ theory of disease, according to which a specific disease is caused by a specific organism. Before this discovery, the common belief, even among health workers, was that diseases were caused by spontaneous generation. In fact, physicians, nurses and caregivers would often neglect the need to wash their hands when moving from one sick patient to another, not realizing that they might be transmitting a disease.

The revolution in medical practice and medications was yet to come when Florence Nightingale began her work in hospitals. Her inquiring mind and methodical approach led her to simple conclusions that she began to apply when working with the sick. Much of the advice she offers in *Notes on Nursing* now seems to be common sense, because the measures she proposes for healthy houses, access to air and light, and sound nutrition are so obviously as effective now as they were in 1859. However, back then not many understood as clearly as she did the link between health and the measures she proposed.

Ms Nightingale stressed that her *Notes* were not a guide to nursing or to becoming a nurse. Her advice was meant to advance and support the work of caregivers in the home. That remains the ambition of this modern edition of her *Notes on Nursing*. Most of the chapters retain the titles she gave them. Each chapter begins with relevant excerpts from the original edition published in 1859; it then updates the information and provides guidance based on the knowledge and developments acquired since that time. The commitment to the caregiver remains the same.

Health of Houses

2

The comfort of home extends beyond its familiarity and amenities. It is, for those assailed by illness or injury, a source of strength and security in a time when both are difficult to retain. But the use of the home as a venue for providing care requires preparation. There are adaptations and additions to the normal home environment that will help make it conducive to the work of the caregiver, and to providing benefits for the patient. The advice offered by Florence Nightingale on the basic steps to making a home a congenial space for caregiving remain applicable today. As with every subsequent chapter in this modern edition, this one begins with an excerpt from the text of the original.

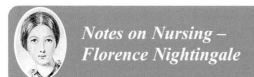

Notes on Nursing –
Florence Nightingale

There are five essential points in securing the health of houses. Without these, no house can be healthy. And it will be unhealthy just in proportion as they are deficient.

Pure air.

Badly constructed houses do for the healthy what badly constructed hospitals do for the sick. Once insure that the air in a house is stagnant, and sickness is certain to follow.

Pure water.

Pure water is more generally introduced into houses than it used to be, thanks to the exertions of the sanitary reformers. This has happily been remedied. But, in many parts of the country, well water of a very impure kind is used for domestic purposes. And when epidemic disease shows itself, persons using such water are almost sure to suffer.

Efficient drainage.

No house with any untrapped drain pipe communicating immediately with a sewer, whether it be from water closet, sink, or gully-grate, can ever be healthy. An untrapped sink may at any time spread fever or pyaemia among the inmates of a palace.

Cleanliness.

Without cleanliness, within and without your house, ventilation is comparatively useless. You cannot have the air of the house pure with dung-heaps under the windows. There are other ways of having filth inside a house besides having dirt in heaps. Old papered walls of years' standing, dirty carpets, uncleansed furniture, are just as ready sources of impurity to the air as if there were a dung-heap in the basement.

Light essential to both health and recovery.

A dark house is always an unhealthy house, always an ill-aired house, always a dirty house. People lose their health in a dark house, and if they get ill they cannot get well again in it.

It is the unqualified result of all my experience with the sick, that second only to their need of fresh air is their need of light; that, after a close room, what hurts them most is a dark room. And that it is not only light but direct sun-light they want. I had rather have the power of carrying my patient about after the sun, according to the aspect of the rooms, if circumstances permit, than let him linger in a room when the sun is off. People think the effect is upon the spirits only. This is by no means the case. The sun is not only a painter but a sculptor. Without going into any scientific exposition we must admit that light has quite as real and tangible effects upon the human body. But this is not all. Who has not observed the purifying effect of light, and especially of direct sunlight, upon the air of a room? The cheerfulness of a room, the usefulness of light in treating disease is all-important.

Aspect, view and sunlight matters of first importance to the sick.

To a sleeper in health it does not signify what the view is from his bed. He ought never to be in it excepting when asleep, and at night. But the case is exactly reversed with the sick, even should they be as many hours out of their beds as you are in yours, which probably they are not. Therefore, that they should be able, without raising themselves or turning in bed, to see out of window from their beds, to see sky and sun-light at least, if you can show them nothing else, I assert to be, if not of the very first importance for recovery, at least something very near it. And you should therefore look to the position of the beds of your sick one of the very first things. If they can see out of two windows instead of one, so much the better. Again, the morning sun and the mid-day sun – the hours when they are quite certain not to be up, are of more importance to them, if a choice must be made, than the afternoon sun. Perhaps you can take them out of bed in the afternoon and set them by the window, where they can see the sun. But the best rule is, if possible, to give them direct sunlight from the moment he rises till the moment he sets.

Another great difference between the bed-room and the sick-room is, that the sleeper has a very large balance of fresh air to begin with, when he begins the night, if his room has been open all day as it ought to be; the sick man has not, because all day he has been breathing the air in the same room, and dirtying it by the emanations from himself. Far more care is therefore necessary to keep up a constant change of air in the sick room.

Infection.

We must not forget what, in ordinary language, is called "Infection;" – a thing of which people are generally so afraid that they frequently follow the very practice in regard to it which they ought to avoid. Nothing used to be considered so infectious or contagious as small-pox; and people not very long ago used to cover up patients with heavy bed clothes, while they kept up large fires and shut the windows. Small-pox, of course, under this regime, is very "infectious." People are somewhat wiser now in their management of this disease. They have ventured to cover the patients lightly and to keep the windows open; and we hear much less of the "infection" of small-pox than we used to do. But do people in our days act with more wisdom on the subject of "infection" in fevers – scarlet fever, measles, &c. – than their forefathers did with small-pox? Does not the popular idea of "infection" involve that people should take greater care of themselves than of the patient? that, for instance, it is safer not to be too much with the patient, not to attend too much to his wants?

True nursing ignores infection, except to prevent it. Cleanliness and fresh air from open windows, with unremitting attention to the patient, are the only defence a true nurse either asks or needs. Wise and humane management of the patient is the best safeguard against infection.

Bedrooms almost universally foul.

During sleep, the human body, even when in health, is far more injured by the influence of foul air than when awake.

Why can't you keep the air all night, then, as pure as the air without in the rooms you sleep in? But for this, you must have sufficient outlet for the impure air you make yourselves to go out; sufficient inlet for the pure air from without to come in. You must have open chimneys, open windows, or ventilators; no close curtains round your beds; no shutters or curtains to your windows, none of the contrivances by which you undermine your own health or destroy the chances of recovery of your sick.

Always air your room, then, from the outside air, if possible. Windows are made to open; doors are made to shut – a truth which seems extremely difficult of apprehension. I have seen a careful nurse airing her patient's room through the door, near to which were two gaslights, (each of which consumes as much air as eleven men,) a kitchen, a corridor, the composition of the atmosphere in which consisted of gas, paint, foul air, never changed, full of effluvia, including a current of sewer air from an ill-placed sink, ascending in a continual stream by a well-staircase, and discharging themselves constantly into the patient's room. The window of the said room, if opened, was all that was desirable to air it. Every room must be aired from without – every passage from without.

Airing damp things in a patient's room.

In laying down the principle that the first object of the nurse must be to keep the air breathed by her patient as pure as the air without, it must not be forgotten that everything in the room which can give off effluvia, besides the patient, evaporates itself into his air. And it follows that there ought to be nothing in the room, excepting him, which can give off effluvia or moisture. Out of all damp towels, &c., which become dry in the room, the damp, of course, goes into the patient's air. Yet this "of course" seems as little thought of, as if it were an obsolete fiction. How very seldom you see a nurse who acknowledges by her practice that nothing at all ought to be aired in the patient's room, that nothing at all ought to be cooked at the patient's fire! Indeed the arrangements often make this rule impossible to observe.

If the nurse be a very careful one, she will, when the patient leaves his bed, but not his room, open the sheets wide, and throw the bed-clothes back, in order to air his bed. And she will spread the wet towels or flannels carefully out upon a horse, in order to dry them.

Effluvia from excreta.

Even in health people cannot repeatedly breathe air in which they live with impunity, on account of its becoming charged with unwholesome matter from the lungs and skin. In disease where everything given off from the body is highly noxious and dangerous, not only must there be plenty of ventilation to carry off the effluvia, but everything which the patient passes must be instantly removed away, as being more noxious than even the emanations from the sick.

Chamber utensils without lids.

The use of any chamber utensil without a lid should be utterly abolished, whether among the sick or well. You can easily convince yourself of the necessity of this absolute rule, by taking one with a lid, and examining the under side of that lid. It will be found always covered, whenever the utensil is not empty, by condensed offensive moisture. Where does that go, when there is no lid?

Earthenware, or if there is any wood, highly polished and varnished wood, are the only materials fit for patients' utensils. The very lid of the old abominable close-stool is enough to breed a pestilence. It becomes saturated with offensive matter, which scouring is only wanted to bring out. I prefer an earthenware lid as being always cleaner. But there are various good new-fashioned arrangements.

Fumigations.

Let no one ever depend upon fumigations, "disinfectants," and the like, for purifying the air. The offensive thing, not its smell, must be removed. A celebrated medical lecturer began one day, "Fumigations, gentlemen, are of essential importance. They make such an abominable smell that they compel you to open the window." I wish all the disinfecting fluids invented made such an "abominable smell" that they forced you to admit fresh air. That would be a useful invention.

Preparing the house

The patient and the caregiver will both benefit from adaptations which are made in the household to accommodate an illness, weakness or disability. Although each situation determines the specific measures to take, there are some basic approaches that suit most circumstances. The home environment in which a patient will live and move needs to be as safe, hygienic and pleasant as possible.

As a general rule, the living space for the patient should be on one floor. It should contain only the furniture that is necessary, and this should be disposed for the convenience of the patient. Once you have positioned the furniture in such a way as to facilitate movement and access by the patient, do not make any arbitrary changes without consulting the patient. Consider adding railings to areas where extra support might be needed, especially if there are staircases. For patients whose eyesight is failing, the use of light and color contrasts in their living space can help them navigate around obstacles.

Once again, the patient should be consulted for these arrangements to make sure they are effective.

If the patient suffers from a respiratory condition such as asthma, emphysema or bronchitis, there are specific measures that should be taken to make the house comfortable. The use of an air conditioner and humidifier offers many benefits. However, it is important to clean the ducts, outlets and air filters of these appliances regularly to ensure they do not aggravate the patient's conditions. Another obvious factor to be avoided is tobacco smoke from visitors. Also, it is best to forego the use of wool blankets and clothing; remove rugs because they are more difficult to clean than tile or other smooth surfaces, and they can also be the cause of slips and falls.

The house should be organized to help the patient maintain body temperature within a normal range. This can be aided by the use of air-conditioning and electric fans, and by the kind of clothing worn by the patient. Healthy individuals can move from an unpleasantly cold or warm room or go in or out of doors. Sickness limits this freedom. As a result, a patient may feel at the mercy of those who condition their environment and may suffer psychologically as well as physically from living in a draughty, cold, humid or overheated space. A patient's ailment or condition will determine susceptibility to feelings of overheating and cold. A room that is comfortable for the caregiver may not be so for the patient. A caregiver should not hesitate to discuss this with a patient, even though some patients will be reluctant to appear to be complaining. The caregiver must always have in mind that the best approach is one that makes the house and the rooms used by the patient as congenial, practical and comfortable as possible.

The bedroom

The bedroom will be the center and limit of the patient's world for long periods of time. It should be made as bright

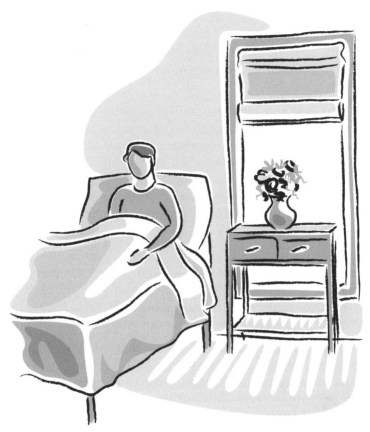

Figure 2.1
The bedroom should ideally be bright and cheerful, with the bed preferably near a window

and as cheerful as possible, with adaptations and decoration that are pleasing for the patient (Figure 2.1). It will also be where much of the work done by the caregiver is carried out, so it needs to be organized practically as well. The caregiver should consult with the patient to make the bedroom as familiar and comfortable as possible. This will include 'personal' touches, such as the placement of art and family photographs so they are clearly visible. Be careful, however, not to clutter the room so much that movement is restricted or impaired. There should be plenty of fresh air available, through windows or doors. The adjustments for heating or air conditioning should be easily accessible.

The bed and mattress need to be solid and narrow so you can reach the patient from either side. Place the bed in an open space, preferably near a window. Make sure it is solid and will not move when leaned on. Place a sturdy chair or table next to the bed to help you get the patient in and out. Acquiring a special, adjustable bed may be necessary in some cases, or special equipment may be required, as discussed later.

The room should be as open to sunlight as possible, both for reasons of health as well as for the patient's morale. However, blinds or shades should be available to darken the room when needed. If possible, these should be useable by the patient when the caregiver is not available.

There are many modern devices that can complement the arrangement of a room, contributing to the patient's sense of security and facilitating the work of the caregiver. An electronic device to monitor the sleep of a patient without having to cause a disturbance by entering the room will be useful in some cases. Long days spent in the same room can be made more agreeable by keeping a supply of books and magazines in the room, according to the patient's preferences. Depending on the condition of the patient, a TV can be installed with a remote control. The patient may enjoy listening to a radio, also equipped with a remote control if possible. For someone who is physically capable of working with a computer, it is possible to accommodate this by installing a PC or by using a laptop computer, preferably equipped with access to the Internet and to email.

The telephone will often be the patient's main access to people outside, including friends and family members. If possible, make this a portable phone – either a mobile telephone or a wireless handset. You may want to position more than one handset in the patient's living space, placing a second phone in the bathroom, for example. A list of personal and emergency numbers should be available for use by the patient or the caregiver. The most important numbers can be programmed for speed dialing using a single number.

The bathroom   ● ● ●

Make sure the path the patient will take from the bed to the bathroom is as direct as possible and that it is clear of any obstructions. Sinks and bathtubs should have railings or grab bars that are positioned for ease of use, and which are suitable for the patient's physical condition and dimensions. Depending on the patient's condition it may be best to remove the lock from the bathroom door.

A shower should be made easy to access and, depending on the condition of the patient, it will be better to have a plastic shower curtain rather than breakable glass doors. Here, again, a grab bar should be installed. Any mats used in the shower or in a bathtub should be of the non-slip variety and cleaned and replaced regularly.

Hand washing   ● ● ●

One of the most effective measures to reduce the risk of infection in the patient's living area is to encourage frequent washing of hands. Contaminated hands represent a danger for the patient and the caregiver, as well as for family members and friends with whom the caregiver and the patient may have contact through the hands.

Hand washing can be done quickly and effectively by following some simple procedures. There are very effective liquid products available for disinfecting hands. It is simple to have these available and to encourage their use by everyone, including the patient.

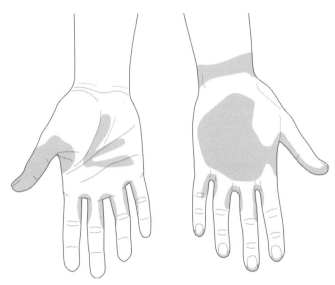

Figure 2.2

Areas of the hand where infection can concentrate

In the absence of such products, hot water is best for washing hands, as it opens up the pores of the skin to remove microorganisms. More detail on hand washing is provided in the Chapter 6.

Medical equipment ● ● ●

Caring for someone can be a daunting physical strain, which modern equipment can make less demanding. Medical devices have been devised to deal with many situations for working with patients who are handicapped, incapacitated or have special needs. You should consult the nurse or physician about equipment that will facilitate your work as a caregiver, and will contribute to the health, mobility and morale of the patient. These can include a wheelchair, devices for lifting and shifting patients in bed, bedpans, mechanical or electrical chairs, a portable commode chair, bath benches, over-the-bed table, walking stand, a cane or crutches. Many of these devices will help the patient feel less dependent, and will also help ensure the caregiver's safety and well-being.

Home first aid kit ● ● ●

The daily activities carried out by a caregiver on behalf of a patient are carefully planned and often repetitive. But accidents happen even in the most organized circumstances. The best recourse will always be to call on professionals in case of a serious accident. Some situations, however, require immediate intervention by the caregiver, using medical supplies that are normally found in a first aid kit. Although many varieties of kits are available commercially, it is often best to assemble one that is adapted to specific circumstances and patients. The kit should be organized in such a way that, in an emergency, anyone can quickly ascertain its contents and make use of them. A basic kit should include:

- A list of everything in the kit.
- List of medications being taken by the patient.
- Band-aids of different sizes and uses.
- Disinfectant solution for cleaning wounds and scrapes.
- An antibiotic ointment.
- Disposable gloves.
- Eye cup and eye pads.
- Face masks.
- Rolled gauze and sterile gauze bandages.
- Elastic bandages.
- Scissors.
- Tweezers.

- Needle.
- Thermometer.
- Tongue depressors.

The kit should be assembled in a box or malleable bag that is easy to find, move and open. It should be left in a clearly visible place, in the bedroom or the bathroom. The patient should be made familiar with the contents of the kit, and its exact location. Any instructions left by the caregiver for someone providing care as a replacement should include information about the first aid kit.

Petty Management

Much of Florence Nightingale's approach to nursing, and to life in general, was based on perceptive planning and good management – what she called being 'in charge'. In *Notes on Nursing* this became the chapter on 'petty management', meaning the organization of details which would help ensure that care was provided efficiently and in a consistent manner. While the focus of her advice was on the most important aspects of care, she shared with readers what she had learned from long experience about the need to go beyond this to an understanding of the patient's mentality, because this would enable the caregiver to be attentive to secondary aspects of care that might also contribute to well-being and recovery. These could range from decorating the bedroom with flowers and plants, depending on the patient's condition, or recognizing the soothing effect on patients of household pets. She also stressed the absolute necessity for a caregiver to foresee periods of regular rest from caregiving, by ensuring that others could take over their responsibilities. Again, this required planning to ensure the replacement is able to assume responsibility for all essential aspects of the patient's plan of care. This last element has become more important with the advent of new medications and methods of treatment. The development of a care plan is the first, essential step for a successful program of care. It is dealt with in this modern edition in the following section in this chapter.

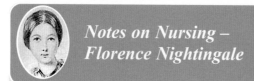

Notes on Nursing – Florence Nightingale

All the results of good nursing, as detailed in these notes, may be spoiled or utterly negatived by one defect, viz.: in petty management, or in other words, by not knowing how to manage that what you do when you are there, shall be done when you are not there. The most devoted friend or nurse cannot be always there. Nor is it desirable that she should. And she may give up her health, all her other duties, and yet, for want of a little management, be not one-half so efficient as another who is not one-half so devoted, but who has this art of multiplying herself – that is to say, the patient of the first will not really be so well cared for, as the patient of the second.

It is as impossible in a book to teach a person in charge of the sick how to manage, as it is to teach her how to nurse. Circumstances must vary with each different case. But it is possible to press upon her to think for herself: Now what does happen during my absence? I am obliged to be away on Tuesday. But fresh air, or punctuality is not less important to my patient on Tuesday than it was on Monday. Or: At 10 P.M. I am never with my patient; but quiet is of no less consequence to him at 10 than it was at 5 minutes to 10.

Curious as it may seem, this very obvious consideration occurs comparatively to few, or, if it does occur, it is only to cause the devoted friend or nurse to be absent fewer hours or fewer minutes from her patient – not to arrange so as that no minute and no hour shall be for her patient without the essentials of her nursing.

Delivery and non-delivery of letters and messages.

An agitating letter or message may be delivered, or an important letter or message not delivered; a visitor whom it was of consequence to see, may be refused, or one whom it was of still more consequence to not see may be admitted – because the person in charge has never asked herself this question, What is done when I am not there?

At all events, one may safely say, a nurse cannot be with the patient, open the door, eat her meals, take a message, all at one and the same time. Nevertheless the person in charge never seems to look the impossibility in the face. Add to this that the attempting this impossibility does more to increase the poor patient's hurry and nervousness than anything else.

Partial measures such as "being always in the way" yourself, increase instead of saving, the patient's anxiety. Because they must be only partial. It is never thought that the patient remembers these things if you do not. He has not only to think whether the visit or letter may arrive, but whether you will be in the way at the particular day and hour when it may arrive. So that your partial measures for "being in the way" yourself, only increase the necessity for his thought. Whereas, if you could but arrange that the thing should always be done whether you are there or not, he need never think at all about it.

For the above reasons, whatever a patient can do for himself, it is better, i.e. less anxiety, for him to do for himself, unless the person in charge has the spirit of management.

Apprehension, uncertainty, waiting, expectation, fear of surprise, do a patient more harm than any exertion. Remember, he is face to face with his enemy all the time, internally wrestling with him, having long imaginary conversations with him. You are thinking of something else. "Rid him of his adversary quickly," is a first rule with the sick.

For the same reasons, always tell a patient and tell him beforehand when you are going out and when you will be back, whether it is for a day, an hour, or ten minutes. You fancy perhaps that it is better for him if he does not find out your going at all, better for him if you do not make yourself "of too much importance" to him; or else you cannot bear to give him the pain or the anxiety of the temporary separation.

No such thing. You ought to go, we will suppose. Health or duty requires it. Then say so to the patient openly. If you go without his knowing it, and he finds it out, he never will feel secure again that the things which depend upon you will be done when you are away, and in nine cases out of ten he will be right. If you go out without telling him when you will be back, he can take no measures nor precautions as to the things which concern you both, or which you do for him.

In institutions where many lives would be lost and the effect of such want of management would be terrible and patent, there is less of it than in the private house. But in both, let whoever is in charge keep this simple question in her head (not, how can I always do this right thing myself, but) how can I provide for this right thing to be always done? Then, when anything wrong has actually happened in consequence of her absence, which absence we will suppose to have been quite right, let her question still be (not, how can I provide against any more of such absences? which is neither possible nor desirable, but) how can I provide against anything wrong arising out of my absence?

What it is to be "in charge"?

How few men, or even women, understand, either in great or in little things, what it is the being "in charge" – I mean, know how to carry out a "charge." From the most colossal calamities, down to the most trifling accidents, results are often traced (or rather *not* traced) to such want of someone "in charge" or of his knowing how to be "in charge." To be "in charge" is certainly not only to carry out the proper measures yourself but to see that everyone else does so too; to see that no one either wilfully or ignorantly thwarts or prevents such measures. It is neither to do everything yourself nor to appoint a number of people to each duty, but to ensure that each does that duty to which he is appointed.

Again, people who are in charge often seem to have a pride in feeling that they will be "missed," that no one can understand or carry on their arrangements, their system, books, accounts, &c., but themselves. It seems to me that the pride is rather in carrying on a system, in keeping stores, closets, books, accounts, &c., so that anybody can understand and carry them on – so that, in case of absence or illness, one can deliver everything up to others and know that all will go on as usual, and that one shall never be missed.

Noise.

Unnecessary noise, or noise that creates an expectation in the mind, is that which hurts a patient. It is rarely the loudness of the noise, the effect upon the organ of the ear itself, which appears to affect the sick. How well a patient will generally bear, e.g., the putting up of a scaffolding close to the house, when he cannot bear the talking, still less the whispering, especially if it be of a familiar voice, outside his door. There are certain patients, no doubt, especially where there is slight concussion or other disturbance of the brain, who are affected by mere noise. But intermittent noise, or sudden and sharp noise, in these as in all other cases, affects far more than continuous noise – noise with jar far more than noise without. Of one thing you may be certain, that anything which wakes a patient suddenly out of his sleep will invariably put him into a state of greater excitement, do him more serious, aye, and lasting mischief, than any continuous noise, however loud.

Never let a patient be waked out of his first sleep.

Never to allow a patient to be waked, intentionally or
accidentally, is a *sine qua non* of all good nursing. If he is
roused out of his first sleep, he is almost certain to have no
more sleep. It is a curious but quite intelligible fact that, if a
patient is waked after a few hours' instead of a few minutes'
sleep, he is much more likely to sleep again. Because pain, like
irritability of brain, perpetuates and intensifies itself. If you
have gained a respite of either in sleep you have gained more
than the mere respite. Both the probability of recurrence and
of the same intensity will be diminished; whereas both will
be terribly increased by want of sleep. This is the reason why
sleep is so all-important. This is the reason why a patient
waked in the early part of his sleep loses not only his sleep,
but his power to sleep. A healthy person who allows himself
to sleep during the day will lose his sleep at night. But it is
exactly the reverse with the sick generally; the more they
sleep, the better will they be able to sleep.

Noise which excites expectation.

I have often been surprised at the thoughtlessness, (resulting in
cruelty, quite unintentionally) of friends or of Physicians who
will hold a long conversation just in the room or passage
adjoining to the room of the patient, who is either every moment
expecting them to come in, or who has just seen them, and
knows they are talking about him. If he is an amiable patient,
he will try to occupy his attention elsewhere and not to listen –
and this makes matters worse – for the strain upon his attention
and the effort he makes are so great that it is well if he is not
worse for hours after. If it is a whispered conversation in the
same room, then it is absolutely cruel; for it is impossible that
the patient's attention should not be involuntarily strained to
hear. Walking on tip-toe, doing

anything in the room very slowly, are injurious, for exactly the same reasons. A firm light quick step, a steady quick hand are the desiderata; not the slow, lingering, shuffling foot, the timid, uncertain touch. Slowness is not gentleness, though it is often mistaken for such: quickness, lightness, and gentleness are quite compatible. Again, if friends and Physicians did but watch, as Nurses can and should watch, the features sharpening, the eyes growing almost wild, of fever patients who are listening for the entrance from the corridor of the persons whose voices they are hearing there, these would never run the risk again of creating such expectation, or irritation of mind.

Or just outside the door.

I need hardly say that the other common cause, namely, for a physician or friend to leave the patient and communicate his opinion on the result of his visit to the friends just outside the patient's door, or in the adjoining room, after the visit, but within hearing or knowledge of the patient is, if possible, worst of all.

Noise of female dress.

It is, I think, alarming, peculiarly at this time, when the female ink-bottles are perpetually impressing upon us "woman's" "particular worth and general missionariness," to see that the dress of women is daily more and more unfitting them for any "mission," or usefulness at all. It is equally unfitted for all poetic and all domestic purposes. A man is now a more handy and far less objectionable being in a sick room than a woman. Compelled by her dress, every woman now either shuffles or waddles – only a man can cross the floor of a sickroom without shaking it! What is become of woman's light step? – the firm, light, quick step we have been asking for?

Unnecessary noise, then, is the most cruel absence of care which can be inflicted either on sick or well. For, in all these remarks, the sick are only mentioned as suffering in a greater proportion than the well from precisely the same causes. Unnecessary (although slight) noise injures a sick person much more than necessary noise (of a much greater amount).

Patient's repulsion to Nurses who rustle.

All doctrines about mysterious affinities and aversions will be found to resolve themselves very much, if not entirely, into presence or absence of care in these things. A nurse who rustles (I am speaking of Nurses professional and unprofessional) is the horror of a patient, though perhaps he does not know why. The fidget of silk and of crinoline, the rattling of keys, the creaking of stays and of shoes, will do a patient more harm than all the medicines in the world will do him good. The noiseless step of woman, the noiseless drapery of woman, are mere figures of speech in this day. Her skirts (and well if they do not throw down some piece of furniture) will at least brush against every article in the room as she moves.

Again, one nurse cannot open the door without making everything rattle. Or she opens the door unnecessarily often, for want of remembering all the articles that might be brought in at once. A good nurse will always make sure that no door or window in her patient's room shall rattle or creak; that no blind or curtain shall, by any change of wind through the open window be made to flap – especially will she be careful of all this before she leaves her patients for the night. If you wait till your patients tell you, or remind you of these things, where is the use of their having a nurse? There are more shy than exacting patients, in all classes; and many a patient passes a bad night, time after time, rather than remind his nurse every night of all the things she has forgotten.

If there are blinds to your windows, always take care to have them well up, when they are not being used. A little piece slipping down, and flapping with every draught, will distract a patient.

Hurry peculiarly hurtful to the sick.

All hurry or bustle is peculiarly painful to the sick. And when a patient has compulsory occupations to engage him, instead of having simply to amuse himself, it becomes doubly injurious. The friend who remains standing and fidgeting about while a patient is talking business to him, or the friend who sits and proses, the one from an idea of not letting the patient talk, the other from an idea of amusing him, – each is equally inconsiderate. Always sit down when a sick person is talking business to you, show no signs of hurry, give complete attention and full consideration if your advice is wanted, and go away the moment the subject is ended.

How to visit the sick and not hurt them.

Always sit within the patient's view, so that when you speak to him he has not painfully to turn his head round in order to look at you. Everybody involuntarily looks at the person speaking. If you make this act a wearisome one on the part of the patient you are doing him harm. So also if by continuing to stand you make him continuously raise his eyes to see you. Be as motionless as possible, and never gesticulate in speaking to the sick.

Never make a patient repeat a message or request, especially if it be some time after. Occupied patients are often accused of doing too much of their own business. They are instinctively right. How often you hear the person, charged with the request of giving the message or writing the letter, say half an hour afterwards to the patient, "Did you appoint 12 o'clock?" or, "What did you say was the address?" or ask perhaps some much more agitating question – thus causing the patient the effort of memory, or worse still, of decision, all over again.

It is really less exertion to him to write his letters himself. This is the almost universal experience of occupied invalids. This brings us to another caution. Never speak to an invalid from behind, nor from the door, nor from any distance from him, nor when he is doing anything.

These things are not fancy.

These things are not fancy. If we consider that, with sick as with well, every thought decomposes some nervous matter, – that decomposition as well as re-composition of nervous matter is always going on, and more quickly with the sick than with the well, – that, to obtrude abruptly another thought upon the brain while it is in the act of destroying nervous matter by thinking, is calling upon it to make a new exertion, – if we consider these things, which are facts, not fancies, we shall remember that we are doing positive injury by interrupting, by "startling a fanciful" person, as it is called. Alas! it is no fancy.

Interruption damaging to sick.

If the invalid is forced, by his avocations, to continue occupations requiring much thinking, the injury is doubly great. In feeding a patient suffering under delirium or stupor you may suffocate him, by giving him his food suddenly, but if you rub his lips gently with a spoon and thus attract his attention, he will swallow the food unconsciously, but with perfect safety. Thus it is with the brain. If you offer it a thought, especially one requiring a decision, abruptly, you do it a real not fanciful injury. Never speak to a sick person suddenly; but, at the same time, do not keep his expectation on the tiptoe.

And to well.

This rule, indeed, applies to the well quite as much as to the sick. I have never known persons who exposed themselves for

years to constant interruption who did not muddle away
their intellects by it at last. The process with them may be
accomplished without pain. With the sick, pain gives warning
of the injury.

Keeping a patient standing.

Do not meet or overtake a patient who is moving about in order
to speak to him, or to give him any message or letter. You might
just as well give him a box on the ear. I have seen a patient fall
flat on the ground who was standing when his nurse came into
the room. This was an accident which might have happened
to the most careful nurse. But the other is done with intention.
A patient in such a state is not going to the East Indies. If
you would wait ten seconds, or walk ten yards further, any
promenade he could make would be over. You do not know
the effort it is to a patient to remain standing for even a quarter
of a minute to listen to you. If I had not seen the thing done
by the kindest Nurses and friends, I should have thought this
caution quite superfluous.

Patients dread surprise.

Patients are often accused of being able to "do much more
when nobody is by." It is quite true that they can. Unless
Nurses can be brought to attend to considerations of the kind
of which we have given here but a few specimens, a very weak
patient finds it really much less exertion to do things for
himself than to ask for them. And he will, in order to do them,
(very innocently and from instinct) calculate the time his nurse
is likely to be absent, from a fear of her "coming in upon" him
or speaking to him, just at the moment when he finds it quite
as much as he can do to crawl from his bed to his chair, or
from one room to another, or down stairs, or out of doors for a
few minutes. Some extra call made upon his attention at that

moment will quite upset him. In these cases you may be sure that a patient in the state we have described does not make such exertions more than once or twice a day, and probably much about the same hour every day. And it is hard, indeed, if nurse and friends cannot calculate so as to let him make them undisturbed. Remember, that many patients can walk who cannot stand or even sit up. Standing is, of all positions, the most trying to a weak patient.

Everything you do in a patient's room after he is "put up" for the night, increases tenfold the risk of his having a bad night. But, if you rouse him up after he has fallen asleep, you do not risk, you secure him a bad night. One hint I would give to all who attend or visit the sick, to all who have to pronounce an opinion upon sickness or its progress. Come back and look at your patient *after* he has had an hour's animated conversation with you. It is the best test of his real state we know. But never pronounce upon him from merely seeing what he does, or how he looks, during such a conversation. Learn also carefully and exactly, if you can, how he passed the night after it.

Effects of over-exertion on sick.

People rarely, if ever, faint while making an exertion. It is after it is over. Indeed, almost every effect of over-exertion appears after, not during such exertion. It is the highest folly to judge of the sick, as is so often done, when you see them merely during a period of excitement. People have very often died of that which, it has been proclaimed at the time, has "done them no harm."

Remember never to lean against, sit upon, or unnecessarily shake, or even touch the bed in which a patient lies. This is invariably a painful annoyance. If you shake the chair on which he sits, he has a point by which to steady himself, in his feet. But on a bed or sofa, he is entirely at your mercy, and he feels every jar you give him all through him.

Conciseness necessary with sick.

Conciseness and decision are, above all things, necessary with the sick. Let your thought expressed to them be concisely and decidedly expressed. What doubt and hesitation there may be in your own mind must never be communicated to theirs, not even (I would rather say especially not) in little things. Let your doubt be to yourself, your decision to them. People who think outside their heads, the whole process of whose thought appears, like Homer's, in the act of secretion, who tell everything that led them towards this conclusion and away from that, ought never to be with the sick.

Irresolution most painful to them.

Irresolution is what all patients most dread. Rather than meet this in others, they will collect all their data, and make up their minds for themselves. A change of mind in others, whether it is regarding an operation, or re-writing a letter, always injures the patient more than the being called upon to make up his mind to the most dreaded or difficult decision. Farther than this, in very many cases, the imagination in disease is far more active and vivid than it is in health. If you propose to the patient change of air to one place one hour, and to another the next, he has, in each case, immediately constituted himself in imagination the tenant of the place, gone over the whole premises in idea, and you have tired him as much by displacing his imagination, as if you had actually carried him over both places.

Above all, leave the sick room quickly and come into it quickly, not suddenly, not with a rush. But don't let the patient be wearily waiting for when you will be out of the room or when you will be in it. Conciseness and decision in your movements, as well as your words, are necessary in the sick room, as necessary as absence of hurry and bustle. To possess yourself entirely will ensure you from either failing – either loitering or hurrying.

What a patient must not have to see.

If a patient has to see, not only to his own but also to his nurse's punctuality, or perseverance, or readiness, or calmness, to any or all of these things, he is far better without that nurse than with her – however valuable and handy her services may otherwise be to him, and however incapable he may be of rendering them to himself.

Reading aloud.

With regard to reading aloud in the sick room, my experience is, that when the sick are too ill to read to themselves, they can seldom bear to be read to. Children, eye-patients, and uneducated persons are exceptions, or where there is any mechanical difficulty in reading. People who like to be read to, have generally not much the matter with them; while in fevers, or where there is much irritability of brain, the effort of listening to reading aloud has often brought on delirium. I speak with great diffidence; because there is an almost universal impression that it is *sparing* the sick to read aloud to them.

Read aloud slowly, distinctly, and steadily to the sick.

But two things are certain: –If there is some matter which *must* be read to a sick person, do it slowly. People often think that the way to get it over with least fatigue to him is to get it over in least time. They gabble; they plunge and gallop through the reading. There never was a greater mistake. Houdin, the conjuror, says that the way to make a story seem short is to tell it slowly. So it is with reading to the sick. I have often heard a patient say to such a mistaken reader, "Don't read it to me; tell it me." Unconsciously he is aware that this will regulate the plunging, the reading with unequal paces, slurring over one part, instead of leaving it out altogether, if it is unimportant, and mumbling another. If the reader lets his own attention wander, and then stops to read up to himself, or finds he has read the wrong bit, then it is all over with the poor patient's chance of not suffering. Very few people know how to read to the sick; very few read aloud as pleasantly even as they speak. In reading they sing, they hesitate, they stammer, they hurry, they mumble; when in speaking they do none of these things. Reading aloud to the sick ought always to be rather slow, and exceedingly distinct, but not mouthing – rather monotonous, but not sing song – rather loud but not noisy – and, above all, not too long. Be very sure of what your patient can bear.

Never read aloud by fits and starts to the sick.

The extraordinary habit of reading to oneself in a sick room, and reading aloud to the patient any bits which will amuse him or more often the reader, is unaccountably thoughtless. What do you think the patient is thinking of during your gaps of non-reading? Do you think that he amuses himself upon what you have read for precisely the time it pleases you to go on reading to yourself, and that his attention is ready for something else at precisely the time it pleases you to begin reading again? Whether the person thus read to be sick or well, whether he be doing nothing or doing something else while being thus read to, the self-absorption and want of observation of the person who does it, is equally difficult to understand – although very often the read*ee* is too amiable to say how much it hurts him.

Variety a means of recovery.

To any but an old nurse, or an old patient, the degree would be quite inconceivable to which the nerves of the sick suffer from seeing the same walls, the same ceiling, the same surroundings during a long confinement to one or two rooms. The superior cheerfulness of persons suffering severe paroxysms of pain over that of persons suffering from nervous debility has often been remarked upon, and attributed to the enjoyment of the former of their intervals of respite. I incline to think that the majority of cheerful cases is to be found among those patients who are not confined to one room, whatever their suffering, and that the majority of depressed cases will be seen among those subjected to a long monotony of objects about them.

Colour and form means of recovery.

The effect in sickness of beautiful objects, of variety of objects, and especially of brilliancy of colour is hardly at all appreciated. Such cravings are usually called the "fancies" of patients. And often doubtless patients have "fancies," as *e.g.* when they desire two contradictions. But much more often, their (so called) "fancies" are the most valuable indications of what is necessary for their recovery. And it would be well if Nurses would watch these (so called) "fancies" closely. I have seen, in fevers (and felt, when I was a fever patient myself), the most acute suffering produced from the patient (in a hut) not being able to see out of a window, and the knots in the wood being the only view. I shall never forget the rapture of fever patients over a bunch of bright-coloured flowers. I remember (in my own case) a nosegay of wild flowers being sent me, and from that moment recovery becoming more rapid.

This is no fancy.

People say the effect is only on the mind. It is no such thing. The effect is on the body, too. Little as we know about the way in which we are affected by form, by colour, and light, we do know this, that they have an actual physical effect. Variety of form and brilliancy of colour in the objects presented to patients are actual means of recovery. But it must be slow variety, *e.g.*, if you shew a patient ten or twelve engravings successively, ten-to-one that he does not become cold and faint, or feverish, or even sick; but hang one up opposite him, one on each successive day, or week, or month, and he will revel in the variety.

Flowers.

The folly and ignorance which reign too often supreme over the sick-room, cannot be better exemplified than by this. While the nurse will leave the patient stewing in a corrupting atmosphere, the best ingredient of which is carbonic acid; she will deny him, on the plea of unhealthiness, a glass of cut-flowers, or a growing plant. Now, no one ever saw "overcrowding" by plants in a room or ward. And the carbonic acid they give off at nights would not poison a fly. Nay, in overcrowded rooms, they actually absorb carbonic acid and give off oxygen. Cut-flowers also decompose water and produce oxygen gas. It is true there are certain flowers, *e.g.*, lilies, the smell of which is said to depress the nervous system. These are easily known by the smell, and can be avoided.

Effect of body on mind.

Volumes are now written and spoken upon the effect of the mind upon the body. Much of it is true. But I wish a little more was thought of the effect of the body on the mind. You who believe yourselves overwhelmed with anxieties, but are able every day … to take your meals with others in other rooms, &c., &c., you little know how much your anxieties are thereby lightened; you little know how intensified they become to those who can have no change; – how the very walls of their sick rooms seem hung with their cares; how the ghosts of their troubles haunt their beds; how impossible it is for them to escape from a pursuing thought without some help from variety.

A patient can just as much move his leg when it is fractured as change his thoughts when no external help from variety is given him. This is, indeed, one of the main sufferings of sickness; just as the fixed posture is one of the main sufferings of the broken limb.

Help the sick to vary their thoughts.

It is an ever recurring wonder to see educated people, who call themselves Nurses, acting thus. They vary their own objects, their own employments, many times a day; and while nursing (!) some bed-ridden sufferer, they let him lie there staring at a dead wall, without any change of object to enable him to vary his thoughts; and it never even occurs to them, at least to move his bed so that he can look out of window. No, the bed is to be always left in the darkest, dullest, remotest, part of the room.

I think it is a very common error among the well to think that "with a little more self-control" the sick might, if they chose, "dismiss painful thoughts" which "aggravate their disease," &c. Believe me, almost *any* sick person, who behaves decently well, exercises more self-control every moment of his day than you will ever know till you are sick yourself. Almost every step that crosses his room is painful to him; almost every thought that crosses his brain is painful to him: and if he can speak without being savage, and look without being unpleasant, he is exercising self-control.

Suppose you have been up all night, and instead of being allowed to have your cup of tea, you were to be told that you ought to "exercise self-control," what should you say? Now, the nerves of the sick are always in the state that yours are in after you have been up all night. We will suppose the diet of the sick to be cared for. Then, this state of nerves is most frequently to be relieved by care in affording them a pleasant view, a judicious variety as to flowers, and pretty things. Light by itself will often relieve it. The craving for "the return of day," which the sick so constantly evince, is generally nothing but the desire for light, the remembrance of the relief which a variety of objects before the eye affords to the harassed sick mind.

The responsibilities of the caregiver

The aspect of providing care which Florence Nightingale called 'Petty Management' has become more complicated today. The tasks which a caregiver needs to be 'in charge' of can range from organizing a daily program of treatment for the patient, maintaining a working relationship with physicians and other health professionals, and ensuring that the patient retains as much 'quality of life' as possible through a program of exercise and other personal activities.

The caregiver has always needed a good measure of love and compassion to provide effective care. This remains as important as ever, but the complexity of the relationships involved, the variety of treatments and medications available, will thwart even the best-intentioned caregiver who cannot combine personal commitment with an organized, systematic approach to providing care.

Developing a plan of care   ● ● ●

The development of a plan of care is the first, essential step in assuming the role of a caregiver. The plan is a road map that everyone involved in providing care for the patient can consult and utilize. The process of developing and writing down the elements of the plan forces the caregiver and anyone else involved in developing it to give some thought to all the elements of providing care, including consideration for the wishes of the patient and the needs of other members of the patient's family. The patient's involvement in developing the plan is not a courtesy but an essential step to ensure the plan will be followed and that it will be effective. It must, as much as possible, be adapted to the personal preferences, habits and desires of the patient.

A written plan tells all those who may have a role in providing care what actions to take and what sequence to follow in giving care. It provides a measure of assurance that there will be no lapses in the process of providing care, especially when the primary caregiver is absent. The care plan is developed to deal with a specific ailment or condition which follows a normal course of development. This means that the plan must also evolve to account for temporary or continuing changes in the condition of the patient, and the course of treatment prescribed by health professionals. The patient will often be the best guide in determining when changes to the care plan are needed to account for new circumstances or a change in condition, mental or physical.

When a number of changes are indicated, the plan must be re-written. Even a daily revision may be required, as, for example, before and after surgery or hospital treatment. On the other hand, a weekly revision might be adequate for a chronic cardiac patient. Ideally, the plan takes into account the patient's normal habits so that established hours for eating, eliminating, sleeping, etc., are changed no more than necessary.

The care plan becomes the caregiver's daily working tool and schedule. It is based on instructions by the physicians, nurses and other health professionals who are treating the patient, and their assessment of the patient's needs in terms of medications, treatment, and diet. The plan enables the caregiver to map out the procedures to be followed every day so that it becomes routine. It constitutes a schedule and a reminder, which can also be followed by anyone who temporarily replaces the main caregiver. As it evolves, the plan also constitutes a record of the treatment program and the status of the patient.

Elements of the care plan

The written plan and any related papers should be kept as a single document, preferably in a loose-leaf ring binder. The elements of the plan will include:

- Physician's, nurse's and other professionals' instructions – clearly identifying each physician or nurse if many are involved. The contact information for each should accompany the instructions.

- Nature of the disease or ailment.

- Medications, dosage, timing and instructions for administering. Patients often have a number of medications which need to be taken at different times of the day. It is crucial to have a detailed schedule that the caregiver or replacement can use every day. The schedule needs to include the name of the medication, the dose, the frequency and any special instructions – such as to be given with or without food, with or without water.

- Things the patient can and should not do (exercise, nutrition, etc.).

- Special equipment and devices needed to care for the patient and where to find these in the house.

- Dietary recommendations or requirements, along with any special instructions on preparation – no salt, nuts, etc.

- Any special care instructions to deal with specific issues.

- Useful information, including emergency telephone numbers for ambulances, medical services on weekends and holidays, etc.

- Recurring daily activities:
  - Morning,
  - Afternoon,

> Bedtime,
> Meals – times, favorites, etc.,
> Treatments – type and times,
> Personal care – bath, hair, skin, massage,
> Mobility,
> Sensory deficits (hearing, vision, etc.).

- Instructions on caregiving related to the patient's individual ailment and condition.

- In a situation where the patient requires specific types of assistance from the caregiver it is essential to provide details and any instructions on how the assistance should be provided. This can include:

> Helping the patient with respiration,
> Helping the patient with eating and drinking,
> Helping the patient with elimination,
> Helping the patient maintain desirable posture in walking, sitting, and lying; and helping move from one position to another,
> Helping the patient rest and sleep,
> Helping the patient with selection of clothing, with dressing and undressing,
> Helping the patient maintain body temperature within normal range,
> Helping the patient keep body clean and well groomed,
> Helping the patient avoid dangers in the environment; and protecting others from any potential danger from the patient, such as infection,
> Helping the patient communicate with others – to express needs and feelings in cases where the ability to communicate is impaired,
> Helping the patient with religious practices,
> Helping the patient with work, or productive occupation.

Each plan for providing care is an individual document, designed to address the health problems of a specific patient and the plan of treatment to be followed. The following provides guidance on other elements which need to be considered in devising the caregiving plan.

Components of basic care	Conditions always present that affect basic needs	Pathological states (as contrasted with specific diseases) that modify basic needs
Assisting the patient with these functions or providing conditions that will enable him to: • breathe normally • eat and drink adequately • eliminate by all avenues of elimination • move and maintain desirable posture (walking, sitting, lying and changing from one to the other) • sleep and rest • select suitable clothing, dress and undress • maintain body temperature within normal range by adjusting clothing and modifying the environment • keep the body clean and well groomed and protect the integument • avoid dangers in the environment and avoid injuring others • communicate with others in expressing emotions, needs, fears, etc. • worship according to his faith, if applicable • work at something that provides a sense of accomplishment	Age: new born, child, youth, adult, middle aged, aged, and dying Temperament, emotional state, or passing mood: • 'normal' or • euphoric and hyperactive • anxious, fearful, agitated or hysterical, or • depressed and hypoactive Social or cultural status: a member of a family unit with friends and status, or a person relatively alone and/or maladjusted, destitute Physical and intellectual capacity: a) normal weight b) underweight c) overweight d) normal mentality e) sub-normal mentality f) gifted mentality g) normal sense of hearing, sight, equilibrium and touch h) loss of special sense i) normal motor power j) loss of motor power	Marked disturbances of fluid and electrolyte balance including starvation states, pernicious vomiting, and diarrhea Acute oxygen want Shock (including 'collapse' and hemorrhage) Disturbances of consciousness – fainting coma, delirium Exposure to cold and heat causing markedly abnormal body temperatures Acute febrile states (all causes) A local injury, wound and/or infection A communicable condition Pre-operative state Post-operative state Immobilization from disease or prescribed as treatment Persistent or intractable pain (Continued)

Components of basic care	Conditions always present that affect basic needs	Pathological states (as contrasted with specific diseases) that modify basic needs
(Continued) • play, or participate in various forms of recreation • learn, discover, or satisfy the curiosity that leads to 'normal' development and health		

An example of a plan of care   ● ● ●

The following is an example of a caregiving plan. It includes all the usual components of basic home care. Drugs and treatment are not included here, but in practice they would be inserted in the appropriate spaces. A similar plan should be developed to cover the period from 7.00 p.m. to 6.30 a.m. The hypothetical plan below organizes care for a hypothetical young adult man who is confined to bed rest for most of each day.

Hour	April 2008						Nursing care	Suggestions for those giving care
	1	2	3	4	5	6		
7.30 a.m.							May go to bathroom for defecation but is to use urinal in bed at other times	Assist patient in going to bathroom or in using bed pan or urinal
8.00							Patient is able to wash wash face and hands and brush teeth in preparation for breakfast Provide fresh drinking water	Important that patient takes fluids (Continued)

Hour	April 2008						Nursing care	Suggestions for those giving care
	1	2	3	4	5	6		
8.30							Breakfast (General diet) (High vitamin)	Encourage patient to drink about 2,000 c.c. and to keep the written record supplied to him
9.00							Bed bath and daily shave. Patient may help but not to point of fatigue	Encourage patient to describe how he feels and to communicate needs. Note these in the care record book
9.30							Note and report any significant changes in appearance of skin	Make note of these and report them to nurse or physician treating the patient
10.00							Visitors, reading, radio, reading mail, writing letters, cross-word puzzles	Family, friends and minister have been to see patient. Discourage more than two visitors at any one time
10.30							Liquid nourishment if desired	Observe for signs of constipation or diarrhea
11.00								Support in contour adjustable chair
11.30								Encourage good posture when sitting (from weakness or habit patient tends to slump)
12.00 noon							Out of bed for one hour – sitting in chair	Wears flannel robe. See that patient is warm while sitting in chair for lunch
12.30 p.m.							Luncheon	Likes to eat lunch with caregiver or a family member, if possible
1.30								Darken room, open window and put 'sleeping' sign on door
2.00							Rest and sleep	
2.30								Encourage chest expansion and straight spine in bed and frequent change of lying posture
								(Continued)

Hour	April 2008						Nursing care	Suggestions for those giving care
	1	2	3	4	5	6		
3.00							Visitors – recreation as above and as desired	Suggest to suitable visitors that patient enjoys being read to and working puzzles with others
3.30							Provide fresh drinking water, liquid nourishment if desired	Observe for signs of constipation or diarrhea
4.00								
4.30								
5.00								
5.30							Out of bed for one hour – sitting in chair	
6.00							Dinner	Appetite is fair. Note what patient eats and drinks and report inadequate intake
6.30								Make summary progress report daily under 'care giver notes'

Working with physicians, nurses and other health professionals ● ● ●

The health of the patient and of the caregiver both depend on effective communication with the health professionals who are providing treatment for the patient. Physicians and nurses provide the benefit of their learning and their experience in guiding the health of the patient. A caregiver has the responsibility to ensure that what they have to offer in terms of diagnosis, recommended treatment and related advice is well understood. A caregiver should ensure that any questions the patient may have for health professionals are asked and dealt with, even if the questions may at times seem silly or misplaced. It is essential that the guidance or instructions received from a physician or nurse be clearly understood by the caregiver and by the patient.

Another facet of the communications between health professionals and caregivers concerns the condition of the patient. A physician or nurse will measure and evaluate the status of the patient's health using professional methods and experience. But it is most often the case that the caregiver is the sole person capable of observing the condition of the patient day in and day out. The caregiver's observations can be vital elements of information for health professionals in assessing situations and making judgements about the health of the patient. Learning how to communicate effectively with professionals is a skill caregivers need to develop or acquire. The efficacy of the care provided and the well-being of the patient depend upon it.

Discussions with the health professionals

The first meeting by the caregiver with the patient's physician or with a nurse or other health professional has to be prepared in advance so everyone can benefit from the information that will be exchanged. The caregiver should gather relevant information on the medical history of the patient and family. These should be written down in note form. A list of symptoms experienced by the person under care should also be included in the caregiver's notes. Add to the list any relevant observations on the patient, such as appetite or lack of, skin condition, sleeping habits, etc. These may help the physician or other health professional identify, diagnose or monitor the patient's condition. The caregiver should write down questions before the meeting, and discuss these with the patient, who may wish to add to the list.

It is preferable to arrive a few minutes early for the appointment. This will give the administrative staff time to complete forms with information about the patient's health, health insurance and other relevant details.

The physician should be provided with any information of a personal or legal nature pertaining to the patient's health. This could be information about health insurance, or the existence of an advance directive, such as a living will or durable power of attorney. Copies of relevant documents should be provided to the physician, for the record. Likewise, the physician should be informed of any familial, religious or ethnic considerations related to the patient's health and treatment.

The caregiver should ask questions about the physician's practice, such as whether to expect other professionals (nurse practitioners, health specialists, therapists) to participate in the patient's care. The physician should be asked about the patient's specific condition, ailment, illness or injury, and how it may develop. Any emergencies that might arise because of the condition should be discussed and the caregiver should understand clearly what is to be done in such an event, particularly if the situation arises on a weekend or other period when it may not be possible to reach the physician immediately.

The caregiver should take notes during the discussion with the physician, questioning the physician whenever something is not clear and noting the answers. If the physician prescribes tests for the patient, the caregiver should ask the reason for specific tests and how long it will take to obtain results, any preparation required, and how the results will be communicated, whether normal or not.

If treatment for a medical problem is ordered, the caregiver should ask about different options, including their effectiveness and possible side effects. Also, questions should be asked about the specific goals for the selected treatment and how the response to treatment will be followed or monitored.

The caregiver should request an explanation of anything that is not understood and ask for an education sheet or handout on the subject if one is available. Having the physician write out instructions and having the caregiver read those instructions back to the physician at the end of the visit is one way to help clarify communication. It offers the physician the opportunity to correct any miscommunication. The same suggestions apply to a trip to the pharmacy for medications.

The caregiver should refer to the list of symptoms and questions prepared before the visit and ask the physician about anything not covered. If many issues remain, the physician may have to schedule another appointment or may refer the person to another healthcare professional, such as a nurse, pharmacist, or dietician, for further information and education.

After the visit, the caregiver should schedule any recommended follow-up appointments. Any prescriptions should be filled, and any material distributed by the pharmacist about the drug should be read. Finally, the caregiver may want to consider keeping a diary of important aspects of the care to be provided (for example, the caregiver for a person with constant headaches may want to record when headaches occur, their timing and associations, and their response to medication).

Keeping records ● ● ●

Keeping a written record on the patient that includes hospitalizations (dates, location, attending physician's name, diagnoses), a family medical history, and significant medical problems is important, because memory alone is not always accurate, and institutional medical records may be unavailable.

Complicated medical regimens should be written out on one sheet of paper; these can be updated as new events occur and the information changes. Copies of laboratory results are also useful to keep for future reference.

Researching the patient's illness or condition ● ● ●

Once a diagnosis of a patient's condition has been made, the caregiver can find additional information that can help to better understand the ailment, how it affects the patient and signs to look for that can help the health professional assess improvements or deterioration in the condition of the patient. The traditional sources of information, such as libraries, are now supplemented by online resources accessible through the Internet. However, some Internet sources are not reliable in that the information may not have come from or been approved by health specialists. Any site designed to sell products or services while also providing information about a health problem should be treated with skepticism, since the information may be biased, incomplete or inaccurate.

Various national and international organizations dealing with health problems offer sites on specific ailments or on general health issues which can be of value. The precautionary principle should be applied when consulting any information from a source that has not been recommended by a health specialist. Public support groups focused on specific illnesses often offer sites that can be useful; they enable a caregiver to compare experiences and to find suggestions on how to assist patients with the illness, including practical matters such as what equipment works best and where to find it. In some communities, there will be special interest groups, which organize discussion meetings on subjects related to providing care. Local health professionals will usually be aware of such groups.

Medications ● ● ●

The panoply of medications for human use has expanded dramatically since the time of Florence Nightingale. The management of a patient's medications is often one of the most important tasks of the caregiver. A patient with a number of simultaneous problems may follow a course of treatment that includes numerous types of medications. The proper administration of these, including correct dosage, timing and observation of side effects are daily tasks that

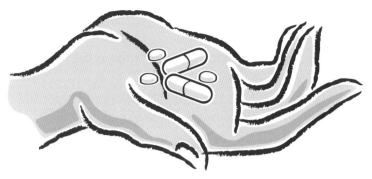

Figure 3.1

Caregivers need to make treatment with medications as safe and effective as possible

the patient is often not able to perform, and for which the caregiver must assume responsibility.

A medication is often defined as a chemical substance intended for use in the diagnosis, cure, relief, treatment or prevention of disease, or intended to affect the structure or function of the body. Medications or drugs are divided into the categories of prescription and non-prescription. Prescription drugs are considered safe for use only under the supervision of a health professional and are dispensed only with a prescription from a licensed individual, such as a physician, dentist, pharmacist, or nurse practitioner. Non-prescription drugs are sold in a variety of commercial outlets and are readily available 'over the counter.' As such they are often referred to as OTCs (over the counter medicines). Regulatory authorities in each country decide how a drug is classified. The label used on the packaging of medications usually includes its chemical name, its generic name, and a proprietary or brand name.

Caregivers can make treatment with medications as safe and effective as possible by the following:

- Ensuring medications are taken exactly as directed, including dosage and timing. Follow any special directions such as taking before meals, with food, not taking alcohol, etc., during the period when a medication is being used.

- Understanding why the medication is being taken and the possible side effects.

- Observing the patient for side effects and reporting any of these to a health professional.

- Consulting a health professional before including non-prescription drugs in a treatment program.

- If the patient has difficulty swallowing medication, consult the physician, nurse or pharmacist for options. Do not improvise by, for example, crushing pills into powder.

- Store the medications in a cool, dry place.

- Get rid of all medications that are no longer being taken or which have expired, as indicated by the manufacturer. The efficacy of medication can diminish over time. It can also become unsafe due to changes in its chemical or physical properties. Be careful to dispose of medications safely. Special care has to be taken that they are not accessible to children. Some medications should not be released into the environment. Consult a pharmacist on the best way to dispose of useless medications.

- Providing the patient with clear information and instructions about medication being taken, and making sure the patient understands.

Medications are introduced into the body by several routes, including orally, by injection into a vein or muscle, under the tongue, by application to the skin, etc. Each route has specific purposes, advantages and disadvantages. However, the method prescribed in each specific case has been selected because it has been found to be the most effective means of having the medication work as it should within the body. Caregivers need to understand and follow the prescribed method of administering the medication. A health professional should be consulted if a caregiver encounters problems administering the medication as prescribed.

Food, other drugs and digestive disorders can affect the absorption of a drug and, therefore, its efficacy. For example, high-fiber foods may bind with a drug and prevent it from being absorbed. Laxatives and diarrhea may reduce drug absorption by speeding up passage through the digestive tract. The length and method of storing a drug can affect its efficacy. The active medication in some products deteriorates and becomes ineffective or harmful if stored improperly or kept too long. Some products must be refrigerated or stored in a cool, dry or dark space. It is important that caregivers closely follow storage directions for medications, and that they are attentive to the expiry date for each medication.

Everyone responds to drugs differently, depending on genetic makeup, age, body size, or the simultaneous use of other drugs. The presence of kidney or liver disease, and the development of tolerance and resistance to a drug also influence its efficacy. Because so many factors affect the response to medications, prescribers choose a drug specifically for an individual patient and adjust the dosage carefully. This process is more complex if the patient takes other medications and has other diseases than the one being treated, because interactions are possible. For some drugs the dose does not have to be adjusted because the same standard dose works well for everyone. The caregiver must always be careful to respect the directions provided for the administration of a medication. To reduce the risk of drug–drug interactions the caregiver should do the following:

- Consult the primary care provider before administering to the patient any new drugs, including OTC non-prescription drugs and dietary supplements, such as medicinal herbs.

- Keep a list of all drugs being taken, and discuss this list periodically with the physician, nurse or pharmacist.

- List all disorders being treated and discuss this as well, periodically, with the physician or nurse.

- Select a pharmacist who provides comprehensive service, including checking for possible interactions, and who maintains a complete medication profile for each patient.

- Inform yourself about the purpose and actions of all medications prescribed.

- Inform yourself about the side effects of all medications prescribed or approved for use, including non-prescription medications. Keep a copy of the medication information on all prescription and OTC medicines to refer to. This information may be provided by the pharmacist and/or inserted in the package you purchase.

- Be certain you know precisely how a medication is to be administered, the time of day when it should be taken, whether it can be taken in the same time period as other medications, and any other requirements.

- Report to the physician, nurse or pharmacist any symptoms you may observe in the patient that might be related to the use of a medication.

- If the patient is seeing more than one primary care practitioner, the caregiver has to ensure that each knows about all the medications being taken.

- The existence of counterfeit drugs has increased in recent years. Any caregiver with doubts about the authenticity of a medication should consult a health professional. Some obvious causes for worry include irregularly shaped or cracked pills, incomplete printing or awkward language on packages, differences in color of the product.

The effects and effectiveness of medications can be altered by food and beverages consumed in the same time period as the medication. Drugs taken orally, for example, must be absorbed through the lining of the stomach or the small intestine. The presence of food in the digestive tract can reduce this absorption, making the medication less effective. This can often be avoided by administering the medication one or two hours after meals. Other drugs, which are irritating, are best given with food, but only certain foods. Therefore, a caregiver has to obtain and follow advice from a professional on such requirements.

Dietary supplements are products that contain a vitamin, mineral, herb or amino acid, and are meant to provide benefits not available solely through a normal diet. Caregivers need to be aware that such supplements may interact with prescription and OTC medications. Before providing any dietary supplements to a patient, the caregiver should discuss this with a health professional.

Drug–disease interactions

Drug–disease interactions most often involve the worsening of a particular disease by a medication used to treat another disease. Such interactions are most common in older individuals, because they are more likely to have more than one disease. A drug taken for a lung disease, for example, may have effects on the heart, and a drug to treat a cold may affect the eyes. This is why it is so important for the caregiver to ensure that all health professionals providing treatment to the patient are aware of all the diseases the patient has and all the medications the patient is taking. Drug–disease interactions are particularly frequent in cases of diabetes, high or low blood pressure, glaucoma and insomnia.

A caregiver needs to be attentive to the possibility that a patient can develop tolerance to a medication; this happens typically when the same medication is used repeatedly over a period of time and the body adapts to its continued presence, making it less effective. Tolerance usually develops because metabolism of the medication speeds up and the number of cell receptors that the medication attaches to, or the strength of the bond, decreases with use. Depending on the degree of tolerance or resistance, the health professional may increase the dosage or recommend a different medication. The caregiver needs to be attentive to any signs that might point to tolerance or resistance, and report them to the health professional.

The regularity with which a patient takes medication, the dosage, and any complicating factors involved in combining medications has to be managed by the caregiver, in consultation with the patient. To assist both in this respect, it is often useful to have recourse to specially designed pill boxes, which the patient can use to take medication as and when prescribed. The caregiver can use the pill box to verify that the medication has been taken as prescribed.

Side effects

Most medications produce several effects besides the 'therapeutic' effect that is wanted for the treatment. Certain antihistamines, for example, cause drowsiness as well as doing the work for which they are taken – to control the symptoms of allergies. Health professionals usually refer to side effects that are unwanted, unpleasant, noxious or potentially harmful by using the term 'adverse drug reaction.' Most adverse drug reactions are mild, and many disappear when the medication is stopped or the dosage is changed. But some adverse drug reactions can be serious and long-lasting. Digestive disturbances – loss of appetite, nausea, a bloating sensation, constipation and diarrhea – are common adverse drug reactions. However, almost any organ system can be affected. In older patients, the brain is commonly affected, resulting in drowsiness and confusion.

Adverse drug reactions may result from an exaggeration of the medication's therapeutic effects. For example, a patient taking a medication to reduce high blood pressure may feel dizzy or light-headed if the medication reduces blood pressure too much. This type of adverse reaction may be due to the dosage of the medication, a particular sensitivity that the patient may have to the medication, or to another medication slowing the metabolism of the first medication, increasing its level in the blood. Some adverse reactions, called 'idiosyncratic reactions,' are simply not well understood. They can include skin rashes, jaundice, anemia, a decrease in white blood cell count, kidney damage, and nerve injury that may impair hearing or sight. Patients who suffer these effects may be allergic or hypersensitive to the medication due to genetic factors that influence how their body metabolizes or responds to the medication.

Some adverse drug reactions are predictable because the mechanisms involved are understood by health professionals. For example, stomach irritation and bleeding may occur in patients who use aspirin or other non-steroidal anti-inflammatory medications. It is known that these medications reduce the production of prostaglandins, which help protect the digestive tract from stomach acid.

There is no scale for establishing the severity of adverse drug reactions, beyond describing them as mild, moderate or severe. Reactions usually considered mild include digestive disturbances, headaches, fatigue, muscle aches and changes in sleep patterns. Even though considered mild, these reactions can be quite disturbing for a patient, who may become less willing to take the medication as instructed.

Moderate reactions can include extensive skin rashes, visual disturbances, muscle tremor, difficulty with urination, and changes in mood or mental function. Mild or moderate reactions do not necessarily mean that a drug will be discontinued, especially if no reliable alternative is available. A health professional may re-evaluate the dosage, frequency of administration, and the timing of doses, for example before or after meals or in the morning rather than at bedtime. Other medications may be used to control adverse drug reactions.

Severe reactions can be life-threatening, such as liver failure or abnormal heart rhythms. Severe reactions are relatively rare but must be dealt with promptly by a health professional when they occur.

Drug allergies

Drug allergies are difficult to anticipate because reactions occur after a patient has been exposed to a medication. The health professional will always inquire if a patient has any known allergies to medication. Allergic reactions vary by individual; they can be minor or life-threatening. Examples are skin rashes and itching, constriction of airways and wheezing, swelling of tissues, which impairs breathing, and a fall in blood pressure to dangerously low levels.

A mild reaction may be treated with an antihistamine, while a severe reaction will require intervention by a health professional. Caregivers need to be attentive to any signs of allergic reaction when a new medication is added to the patient's treatment program. Even mild allergic reactions should be reported to the primary care provider.

Prevention ● ● ●

Preventive care aims to ensure that measures are taken to make certain that the living environment and the care provided contribute to improvements in the patient's condition. One of the most dramatic improvements in preventive medicine over the past decades has been the development of vaccines for infectious diseases, such as diphtheria, pertussis, tetanus, mumps, measles, rubella and polio. Methods for prevention include:

- Vaccinations to prevent infectious diseases.
- Screening program, such as for high blood pressure, diabetes and cancer.
- Chemoprevention, such as aspirin to reduce the risk of heart attacks and strokes.

- Counseling that aims to have individuals make healthy lifestyle choices; for example, about their diet.

The prevention measures recommended for an individual will depend on factors such as age and gender. For example, the pneumonia vaccine is recommended for everyone after age 65 to prevent the most common forms of pneumonia. The caregiver should consult a health professional about preventive measures that can be effective for their patient.

Exercise and fitness

Regular exercise is one of the best things any individual can do to preserve or improve health. Every caregiver should consider adopting a personal exercise program, adapted to the time available and the caregiver's physical condition. Patients should also be encouraged to have a regular period of exercise, adapted to their physical ability and to their treatment program. In some cases, health professionals will recommend that the exercise be supervised by a physical therapist or by an experienced trainer. Such professionals will be able to devise an exercise program that takes into account any special considerations. For example, patients suffering from osteoarthritis should avoid exercise that puts undue stress on joints.

Most people should exercise no more than three to four times per week. Skeletal muscles start to break down when exercised too intensively, which can lead to bleeding and microscopic tearing, which results in muscles feeling sore. Additionally, individuals should vary the way they exercise over time. The body adapts to routine, so that doing the same exercises over time becomes less effective for strength and cardiovascular fitness. Once again, a training professional can devise an exercise program that takes into account all the aspects of a patient's condition, including the need to vary the program over time.

Rehabilitation • • •

Rehabilitation services are needed by individuals who have sustained severe injury due to an accident, a stroke, an infection, a tumor, surgery or progressive disease. Patients whose bodies become weak after prolonged bed rest are also in need of rehabilitation. The type, level and goals of rehabilitation will differ for each patient. For example, the goal for an older patient who has suffered a stroke may be to restore the ability to perform as many self-care activities, such as dressing and eating, as possible. The goal for a younger person who has been in a car accident is often to restore full, unrestricted freedom of movement.

To initiate a formal rehabilitation program, a health professional writes a referral (similar to a prescription) to a physiatrist (a physician who is board-certified in rehabilitation medicine), an occupational or physical therapist, or a rehabilitation center. The referral establishes the goals of therapy, a description of the type of illness or injury, and its date of onset. The referral also specifies the type of therapy needed, such as ambulation training (help with walking) or training in activities of daily life, such as eating, dressing, grooming or toileting.

Where the rehabilitation takes place varies according to the person's needs. Care in a hospital or rehabilitation center may be necessary for people with severe disabilities. In such settings, a rehabilitation team provides care. Along with the physician or therapist, this team may include nurses, psychologists, social workers, other healthcare practitioners and family caregivers.

People who require less care, such as those who can transfer from bed to a chair or from a chair to a toilet, can often obtain rehabilitation services at home from a personal caregiver. This is by far the most desirable form of rehabilitation, but it can be physically and emotionally draining. It may be preferable for a visiting physical therapist, occupational therapist or other healthcare worker to assist the principal caregiver to conduct the rehabilitation program. The caregiver's health is a consideration in making such a decision, since the rehabilitation program should provide benefits to the patient without risking harm to the caregiver.

Helping the patient with respiration ● ● ●

Everyone's health is affected to an important degree by the quality of respiration. It is one of the aspects of a patient's condition to which the caregiver needs to be particularly attentive. There are postures that restrict proper breathing, and others that encourage optimum chest expansion and free use of all the muscles involved in respiration. (A diagram of the respiratory system is shown in Figure 3.2.) The caregiver and the patient should obtain instruction on these postures from a health professional. When patients must be helped to assume such postures, it will be the caregiver's responsibility to know the methods to use to position the patient and to maintain the best posture. This can include selecting the type of bed or chairs that favor these postures, and the use and placement of pillows, pads and rolls to maintain positions that promote normal breathing. The patient should also be made aware of postures that favor respiration.

Inadequate respiration can be occasioned by causes other than poor posture, including emotional stress or obstruction of air passages. A caregiver must observe and communicate to a health professional any signs of difficulty in breathing experienced by a patient. Under some extreme circumstances it may be necessary for the caregiver to intervene. To this end, it is important that the caregiver has obtained some training or instruction from a health professional on the measures that can be taken, and to have the necessary instruments or equipment available. (Emergency tracheotomies performed by lay persons have saved lives.) Since nothing is so threatening to life as a

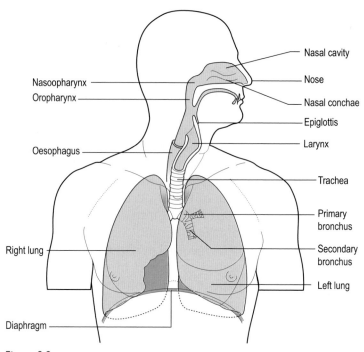

Figure 3.2

The respiratory system

respiratory block, the caregiver of a patient subject to this condition should learn what causes it, how to relieve it and, if possible, how to prevent it. Every caregiver should learn how to give artificial respiration and perform cardiac resuscitation.

Caregivers should be alert to the effects on the patient of environmental factors such as room temperature and humidity, and the presence of irritants in the air. Any problems observed should be discussed with a physician or nurse, who may recommend changes such as the use or discontinuation of air conditioning and humidifiers. For some patients, the only comfortable environment will be an open window or door rather than mechanical devices.

Travelling with a patient   ● ● ●

Facilities for travelling have greatly improved and increased since Florence Nightingale's time, and it is now possible for some patients to travel for pleasure, to follow a course of treatment in another location, or to attend to personal and family matters. The condition of the patient is always the determining factor in their ability to travel; the health professionals who are treating the patient will determine if travel is possible, under what conditions and with which kind of treatment.

The caregiver who plans to travel with a patient needs to be attentive to their own health as well as that of the person being cared for. No matter what the destination, it is always important for the caregiver to assemble a travel kit of appropriate medications and supplies, as prescribed and adapted to the condition of the patient. It is invaluable to have a letter from the physician that summarizes the patient's medical history, the names of medications being taken, dosages and dates of treatment. Proof of health insurance is also important. Verify if the health insurance includes a provision for emergency evacuation.

If the health professional or the caregiver anticipates the need for healthcare at the destination, this should be planned in advance. The caregiver will need to know what type of care might be needed, and will need to determine exactly where it can be found and any special conditions for access to such care. If medications are prescribed, either as part of the regular care plan or as special support during travel, make a detailed list of medications that are to be taken, and the frequency and dosage. Ensure there is more than the quantity absolutely needed of important medications in case there should be delays during travel or an unexpected prolongation of the stay at the destination.

Airlines usually provide special services for patients, but it is important to notify airline staff in advance of any requirements. Airline staff can be available to bring a patient aboard the airplane in a wheelchair and to take them off the plane at the destination. Seating arrangements can also be adapted (aisle or window) depending on the patient's condition and preferences. Special meals are also available if they are requested in advance. The best time to first raise any such requirements is when the flight reservations are being made. The travel agency or airline agent will tell the caregiver what is available and if any further contact needs to be made with travel personnel.

Attention to such details is also important when reserving hotel rooms or ground transportation. If the patient requires assistance entering and leaving a taxi or bus this needs to be mentioned when making arrangements. Hotels can also provide wheelchairs or other special equipment such as ramps, hoists, bathroom bars etc., but it is important to request them in advance, when making the reservation.

Be aware of restrictions on items that can be taken in carry-on luggage and handbags. Have a list of medications, and a note from a physician, with contact numbers, that the patient needs to take these medications. Notify the airline that these medications will be carried on board, and pack them in accordance with the instructions the airline will provide

Medications and travel

Medications should be carried in their original containers so that the precise names and instructions for taking them can be reviewed in an emergency. The generic name of the medication is more useful that its brand name, as the latter can vary between different countries. The caregiver should pack an extra supply of medications in a carry-on bag in case checked-in bags are lost or delayed in transit. The caregiver will need a letter from a physician explaining the medical need for these supplies, which might include items such as opioids, syringes, etc., which would attract the attention of customs officers. In addition, syringes should be packed together with the medications that are dispensed in them. The caregiver should also check in advance with relevant airports, airlines, or embassies to know what additional documentation will be helpful to make travel with these supplies possible.

For travel to another country, verify if the patient's health or other insurance allows for medical evacuation. If so, note telephone numbers and other information (e.g. email address) about contacting the insurer. Record the number of your country's consular services in the country to which you are travelling (these are often only available in the capital city). If the patient has a special condition that might require treatment, be sure to inform the airline. In addition, inform the airline about any special equipment that might be needed and any special meals. If the patient requires assistance boarding and leaving the airplane, notify the travel agent and/or the airline in advance of the trip.

Preventive vaccination may be needed for travel to some countries and regions of the world, such as for hepatitis A and B, polio, yellow fever, etc. Some vaccines take up to 6 months to achieve their maximum effect. For some travel it may be necessary to obtain an International Certificate of Vaccination. The caregiver should consult a health professional about any of these requirements well in advance of any planned travel with the patient.

A caregiver travelling with a patient to some international destinations needs to be very attentive to protect the patient, and themself, from infections that can provoke diarrhea. This can be done by using only water that has been filtered, boiled, chlorinated and, usually, sealed in a bottle. Avoid ice in cold drinks, eat only freshly prepared foods that have been heated to steaming temperatures, eat only fruits and vegetables that can be peeled or shelled, and avoid food sold from street stands. Above all, wash hands frequently. In most cases this type of diarrhea subsides by itself and requires only the regular drinking of fluids to prevent dehydration. If the condition persists it may be necessary to consult a physician or nurse. Information about the health services available at the destination should be part of the advance planning for the trip.

4

Food

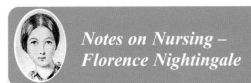

Notes on Nursing –
Florence Nightingale

Taking food.

What of attention to hours of taking food.

Every careful observer of the sick will agree in this that
thousands of patients are annually starved in the midst of
plenty, from want of attention to the ways which alone make
it possible for them to take food. This want of attention is as
remarkable in those who urge upon the sick to do what is quite
impossible to them, as in the sick themselves who will not
make the effort to do what is perfectly possible to them.

For instance, to the large majority of very weak patients it is
quite impossible to take any solid food before 11 A.M., nor
then, if their strength is still further exhausted by fasting till
that hour. For weak patients have generally feverish nights and,
in the morning, dry mouths; and, if they could eat with those
dry mouths, it would be the worse for them. A spoonful of
beef-tea, of arrowroot and wine, of egg flip, every hour, will
give them the requisite nourishment, and prevent them from
being too much exhausted to take at a later hour the solid food,
which is necessary for their recovery. And every patient who
can swallow at all can swallow these liquid things, if he

chooses. But how often do we hear a mutton-chop, an egg, a bit of bacon, ordered to a patient for breakfast, to whom (as a moment's consideration would show us) it must be quite impossible to masticate such things at that hour.

Again, a nurse is ordered to give a patient a tea-cup full of some article of food every three hours. The patient's stomach rejects it. If so, try a table-spoon full every hour; if this will not do, a tea-spoon full every quarter of an hour.

Life often hangs upon minutes in taking food.

If we did but know the consequences which may ensue, in very weak patients, from ten minutes' fasting or repletion (I call it repletion when they are obliged to let too small an interval elapse between taking food and some other exertion, owing to the nurse's unpunctuality), we should be more careful never to let this occur. In very weak patients there is often a nervous difficulty of swallowing, which is so much increased by any other call upon their strength that, unless they have their food punctually at the minute, which minute again must be arranged so as to fall in with no other minute's occupation, they can take nothing till the next respite occurs – so that an unpunctuality or delay of ten minutes may very well turn out to be one of two or three hours. And why is it not as easy to be punctual to a minute? Life often literally hangs upon these minutes.

Food never to be left by the patient's side.

To leave the patient's untasted food by his side, from meal to meal, in hopes that he will eat it in the interval is simply to prevent him from taking any food at all. I have known patients literally incapacitated from taking one article of food after another, by this piece of ignorance. Let the food come at the right time, and be taken away, eaten or uneaten, at the right time; but never let a patient have "something always standing" by him, if you don't wish to disgust him of everything.

On the other hand, I have known a patient's life saved (he was sinking for want of food) by the simple question, put to him by the physician, "But is there no hour when you feel you could eat?" "Oh, yes," he said, "I could always take something at —o'clock and —o'clock." The thing was tried and succeeded. Patients very seldom, however, can tell this; it is for you to watch and find out.

That the more alone an invalid can be when taking food, the better, is unquestionable; and, even if he must be fed, the nurse should not allow him to talk, or talk to him, especially about food, while eating.

When a person is compelled, by the pressure of occupation, to continue his business while sick, it ought to be a rule WITHOUT ANY EXCEPTION WHATEVER, that no one shall bring business to him or talk to him while he is taking food, nor go on talking to him on interesting subjects up to the last moment before his meals, nor make an engagement with him immediately after, so that there be any hurry of mind while taking them.

Upon the observance of these rules, especially the first, often depends the patient's capability of taking food at all, or, if he is amiable and forces himself to take food, of deriving any nourishment from it.

Nurse must have some rule of thought about her patient's diet.

I would say to the nurse, have a rule of thought about your patient's diet; consider, remember how much he has had, and how much he ought to have to-day. Generally, the only rule of the private patient's diet is what the nurse has to give. It is true she cannot give him what she has not got; but his stomach does not wait for her convenience, or even her necessity. If it is used to having its stimulus at one hour to-day, and to-morrow it does not have it, because she has failed in getting it, he will suffer. She must be always exercising her ingenuity to supply defects, and to remedy accidents which will happen among the best contrivers, but from which the patient does not suffer the less, because "they cannot be helped."

One very minute caution, – take care not to spill into your patient's saucer, in other words, take care that the outside bottom rim of his cup shall be quite dry and clean; if, every time he lifts his cup to his lips, he has to carry the saucer with it, or else to drop the liquid upon, and to soil his sheet, or his bed-gown, or pillow, or if he is sitting up, his dress, you have no idea what a difference this minute want of care on your part makes to his comfort and even to his willingness for food.

What food?

Common errors in diet.

I will mention one or two of the most common errors among women in charge of sick respecting sick diet. One is the belief that beef tea is the most nutritive of all articles. Now, just try and boil down a lb. of beef into beef tea, evaporate your beef tea, and see what is left of your beef. You will find that there is barely a teaspoonful of solid nourishment to half a pint of water in beef tea, – nevertheless there is a certain reparative quality in it, we do not know what, as there is in tea, – but it may safely be given in almost any inflammatory disease, and is as little to be depended upon with the healthy or convalescent where much nourishment is required. Again, it is an ever ready saw that an egg is equivalent to a lb. of meat, – whereas it is not at all so.

Eggs.

Also, it is seldom noticed with how many patients, particularly of nervous or bilious temperament, eggs disagree. All puddings made with eggs, are distasteful to them in consequence. An egg, whipped up with wine, is often the only form in which they can take this kind of nourishment.

Meat without vegetables.

Again, if the patient has attained to eating meat, it is supposed that to give him meat is the only thing needful for his recovery; whereas scorbutic sores have been actually known to appear among sick persons living in the midst of plenty in England, which could be traced to no other source that this, viz.: that the nurse, depending on meat alone, had allowed the patient to be without vegetables for a considerable time, these latter being so badly cooked that he always left them untouched.

Observation, not chemistry, must decide sick diet.

In the great majority of cases, the stomach of the patient is guided by other principles of selection than merely the amount of carbon or nitrogen in the diet.

The main question is what the patient's stomach can assimilate or derive nourishment from, and of this the patient's stomach is the sole judge. Chemistry cannot tell this. The patient's stomach must be its own chemist. The diet which will keep the healthy man healthy, will kill the sick one. The same beef which is the most nutritive of all meat and which nourishes the healthy man, is the least nourishing of all food to the sick man, whose half-dead stomach can *assimilate* no part of it, that is, make no food out of it. On a diet of beef tea healthy men on the other hand speedily lose their strength.

Sound observation has scarcely yet been brought to bear on sick diet.

To watch for the opinions, then, which the patient's stomach gives, rather than to read "analyses of foods," is the business of all those who have to settle what the patient is to eat – perhaps the most important thing to be provided for him after the air he is to breathe. I should therefore say that incomparably the most important office of the nurse, after she has taken care of the patient's air, is to take care to observe the effect of his food, and report it to the health attendant.

Helping the patient with eating and drinking

There is no more important element in the preparation for being a caregiver than to understand the critical nature of nutrition for a patient who is ill or injured. When patients are incapacitated for an extended period of time their emotional state may affect nutrition, either because of changes in appetite or capricious selection of food. Immobilization of a bedfast patient or defects in digestion, absorption or metabolism can contribute to poor utilization of food. The presence of infections, wounds, fractures or anemias may increase the requirements for various nutrients above the normal levels and require additions to the usual diet to meet these needs. For both the obese and the underweight patient, the need to achieve the desirable weight is frequently an essential step in rehabilitation. The individual who has problems with chewing or swallowing needs modifications in consistency of food to maintain an adequate diet. Therapeutic diets are frequently prescribed as part of the treatment for diabetes, cardiac disease, gastro-intestinal disorders, liver or gallbladder disease, and other medical conditions.

While the physician, nurse or nutritionist prescribe the diet of a patient, it is the caregiver who can best ensure that food and drink are taken properly. Lifetime food habits based on the cultural, social and economic background of the family, and individual idiosyncrasies are difficult to

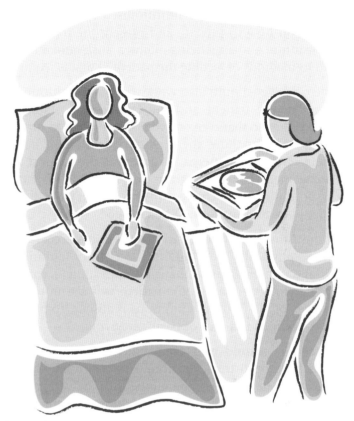

Figure 4.1

Nutrition is critical for a patient who is ill or injured, and enjoyment of meals will aid recovery

change. The caregiver has the opportunity to note what food the patient likes or does not like, and to report these observations to a nutritionist, who can use the information as input when prescribing a diet that best meets the nutritional requirements of the patient, while also respecting preferences as much as possible. The caregiver needs to be attentive to all aspects of food. Any concerns such as strong aversions, allergies or cultural taboos must be communicated to the nurse and nutritionist. The caregiver should discuss the diet with the nutritionist, to understand the basis for their recommendations. A nutritionist can also provide guidance on how to prepare and present the food in the most healthful and appetizing manner. Such guidance can extend to methods of feeding the patient, if that is required.

The caregiver should also work with the nutritionist to ensure that the patient and the family understand the prescribed diet, so that everyone will be motivated to support the patient in making the changes required in eating patterns. Once new patterns are accepted, the support and encouragement of the caregiver are often needed if they are to continue. With changes in the patient's condition, the diet plan, too, must often be changed.

If the patient is prepared for eating in his accustomed manner, physically comfortable, free from emotional stress, and if the meal is aesthetically appealing (according to the patient's standards), the patient will eat more than if any one, or all, of these conditions is absent. To provide these conditions is a part of basic caregiving.

Caregivers should only feed patients when all other options have been tried and found to be impractical. In some circumstances it will be enough for the caregiver to spend time with the patient at mealtimes to encourage independence in taking food. Being able to eat and enjoy a meal unaided is part of recovery for a patient, in terms of both physical and mental health.

Feeding ill and handicapped persons ● ● ●

Very ill or handicapped persons are often unable to feed themselves. In such cases, caregivers must feed them or arrange with family, friends or qualified volunteer workers to do so. It should be borne in mind, however, that it is psychologically difficult for patients that this most intimate of activities, taking food, has to be done for them by someone else. It can also be taxing for the caregiver to feed a sick or injured patient. The caregiver should seek guidance from a nutritionist about feeding the patient. This will help reduce any anxiety or frustrations the caregiver may experience when having to feed the patient, and will contribute to the well-being of both.

It should not be assumed that mealtime will by itself constitute a pleasurable moment for everyone, especially a patient who has to be fed. And unless it is a pleasure, unless the patient finds the food appetizing, and feels that the caregiver who is serving the food does it gladly, the meal is likely to be eaten quickly or partially in order to get it over with.

A caregiver must create an atmosphere that is comfortable for the patient, and for themself. A caregiver who is feeding a patient should be comfortably seated, if at all possible, and the food placed so that both patient and caregiver can see the tray or table. The patient should be encouraged to assume responsibility for eating, even if it is only for part of a meal. The ability of a patient to resume a normal and important activity such as eating contributes to regaining a sense of independence and health. There is more continuity in the patient's rehabilitation if the same caregiver feeds the patient every day. This is also preferable for continuity in noting changes in the patient's appetite or willingness and ability to take food. A patient who is sick at home should be encouraged to go to the family table as soon as privacy and quiet cease to be demanded by his condition. Everything that can be done to increase the pleasurable aspects of eating will help the patient, especially when their appetite is not normal. Someone who is already ill or convalescing is especially susceptible to the adverse effects of food that may have been poorly prepared or stored.

Under certain circumstances, patients require extra-oral feedings. Some extra-oral feedings need to be attended by trained health professionals, while others can be handled by the caregiver following training. The caregiver should learn about the principles of the various therapies.

Washing hands ● ● ●

Washing hands before meals is a basic rule of personal hygiene, which becomes even more important for a patient and all those who have a 'hand' in providing food for the patient. Human hands carry and transmit microorganisms, which means that frequent hand washing is an especially important means for preventing infection. Caregivers should develop the habit of washing hands frequently, using soap or special solutions. Everyone with a role in providing food for the patient should follow the same rule, including friends or relatives who may occasionally come to eat with the patient, or assist the patient in eating. This is one of the single most important measures a caregiver can take to protect everyone involved against infection.

To facilitate hand washing, the caregiver can make sure the eating area has a supply of hand-washing solution. If none is available, hand washing can be done quickly and effectively by following some simple procedures. Hot water is best for washing hands, as it opens up the pores of the skin to remove microorganisms. Cuts, abrasions and skin lesions on the hands of a caregiver can be a source of infection. In such cases, in addition to washing hands, the caregiver or anyone else assisting with feeding the patient should wear disposable gloves.

There are some additional points to keep in mind for the preparation and serving of food to a patient:

- The caregiver must follow closely any special diet devised by a nutritionist or other health specialist; however, the caregiver should take note of any dislikes or reactions to this diet by the patient and report them. This should always include any preferences expressed by the patient, since these may change over time.

- Always disinfect any kitchen surface used to prepare food, such as a counter or chopping board and sink, with a bleach solution (1 tsp chlorine bleach per litre of water) on a regular basis.

- Wash hands with antibacterial soap before preparing food and dry them with a clean towel of paper or cotton.

- Fish and red meat should be cooked thoroughly, especially any meat or fish that has been chopped or ground into patties or sticks.

- All vegetables and fruits that are not thoroughly cooked should be carefully washed.

- The patient's condition or habits may dictate serving meals at other than regular times. A nutritionist can provide advice, and the patient should be consulted about preferences for eating time and about degrees of hunger felt at different times of the day.

- In consulting a nurse, physician or nutritionist about the patient's diet, the caregiver needs to understand clearly if there are restrictions on specific foods, condiments or seasonings, such as sugar, salt, potassium, and other normal ingredients.

- The patient should be encouraged to drink regularly, inkeeping with any special guidance established by a health professional.

- Encourage the patient to eat in a separate dining area, away from the sleeping and resting area.

- Encourage patients to invite friends and family to share a meal, as the patient's condition permits. No meal is as enjoyable for someone confined by illness than one shared with relatives and friends.

- Ensure equipment, such as bedpans and commodes, is removed from the eating area.

- Ensure hands are washed beforehand.

- Ensure the mouth is rinsed before the meal, and clean dentures if necessary.

- If the patient takes food in bed, it should be in a comfortable sitting position, with the table or tray at the correct height and the food within easy reach.

- Provide appropriate dishes and cutlery.

- Ensure food is served at the correct temperature. A cold plate is unpalatable, especially for patients whose pleasures are often limited to meals.

Eating aids

A physician or nurse can advise the caregiver in cases where the patient's difficulties in eating or drinking can be eased through the use of special dishes or utensils. Many such devices have been produced, including: specially shaped spoons for patients who cannot easily flex their wrists; cups with a cover, a spout or two handles and a suction base; food-warming dishes for slow eaters; and utensils with special grip handles. Once again, a nutritionist or other health professional will know what is available to deal with a particular condition and which of these numerous implements is best for the individual circumstances.

Bed and Bedding

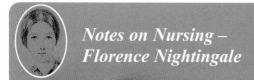

Notes on Nursing –
Florence Nightingale

Bed and bedding.

A few words upon bedsteads and bedding; and principally as regards patients who are entirely, or almost entirely, confined to bed.

Uncleanliness of ordinary bedding.

If I were looking out for an example in order to show what not to do, I should take the specimen of an ordinary bed in a private house: a wooden bedstead, two or even three mattresses piled up to above the height of a table; a vallance attached to the frame – nothing but a miracle could ever thoroughly dry or air such a bed and bedding. The patient must inevitably alternate between cold damp after his bed is made, and warm damp before, both saturated with organic matter, and this from the time the mattresses are put under him till the time they are picked to pieces, if this is ever done.

Air your dirty sheets, not only your clean ones.

If you consider that an adult in health exhales by the lungs and skin in the twenty-four hours three pints at least of moisture, loaded with organic matter ready to enter into putrefaction; that in sickness the quantity is often greatly increased, the quality is always more noxious – just ask yourself next where does all this moisture go to? Chiefly into the bedding, because it cannot go anywhere else. And it stays there; because, except perhaps a weekly change of sheets, scarcely any other airing is attempted. A nurse will be careful to fidgetiness about airing the clean sheets from clean damp, but airing the dirty sheets from noxious damp will never even occur to her. Besides this, the most dangerous effluvia we know of are from the excreta of the sick – these are placed, at least temporarily, where they must throw their effluvia into the underside of the bed, and the space under the bed is never aired; it cannot be, with our arrangements. Must not such a bed be always saturated, and be always the means of re-introducing into the system of the unfortunate patient who lies in it, that excrementitious matter to eliminate which from the body nature had expressly appointed the disease?

Bed not to be too wide.

There is a prejudice in favour of a wide bed – I believe it to be a prejudice. All the refreshment of moving a patient from one side to the other of his bed is far more effectually secured by putting him into a fresh bed; and a patient who is really very ill does not stray far in bed. But it is said there is no room to put a tray down on a narrow bed. No good nurse will ever put a tray on a bed at all. If the patient can turn on his side, he will eat more comfortably from a bed-side table; and on no account whatever should a bed ever be higher than a sofa. Otherwise the patient feels himself "out of humanity's reach;" he can get at nothing for himself; he can move nothing for himself. If the patient cannot turn, a table over the bed is a better thing. I need hardly say that a patient's bed should never have its side against the wall. The nurse must be able to get easily to both sides of the bed, and to reach easily every part of the patient without stretching – a thing impossible if the bed be either too wide or too high.

Bed not to be too high.

When I see a patient in a room nine or ten feet high upon a bed between four and five feet high, with his head, when he is sitting up in bed, actually within two or three feet of the ceiling, I ask myself, is this expressly planned to produce that peculiarly distressing feeling common to the sick, viz., as if the walls and ceiling were closing in upon them, and they becoming sandwiches between floor and ceiling, which imagination is not, indeed, here so far from the truth? If, over and above this, the window stops short of the ceiling, then the patient's head may literally be raised above the stratum of fresh air, even when the window is open.

If a bed is higher than a sofa, the difference of the fatigue of getting in and out of bed will just make the difference, very often, to the patient (who can get in and out of bed at all) of being able to take a few minutes' exercise, either in the open air or in another room. It is so very odd that people never think of this, or of how many more times a patient who is in bed for the twenty-four hours is obliged to get in and out of bed than they are, who only, it is to be hoped, get into bed once and out of bed once during the twenty-four hours.

Nor in a dark place.

A patient's bed should always be in the lightest spot in the room; and he should be able to see out of the window.

Bed sores.

It may be worthwhile to remark, that where there is any danger of bed-sores a blanket should never be placed *under* the patient. It retains damp and acts like a poultice.

Heavy and impervious bed clothes.

Never use anything but light Whitney blankets as bed covering for the sick. The heavy cotton impervious counterpane is bad, for the very reason that it keeps in the emanations from the sick person, while the blanket allows them to pass through. Weak patients are invariably distressed by a great weight of bed clothes, which often prevents their getting any sound sleep whatever.

NOTE – One word about pillows. Every weak patient, be his illness what it may, suffers more or less from difficulty in breathing. To take the weight of the body off the poor chest, which is hardly up to its work as it is, ought therefore to be the object of the nurse in arranging his pillows. Now what does she do and what are the consequences? She piles the pillows one-a-top of the other like a wall of bricks. The head is thrown upon the chest. And the shoulders are pushed forward, so as not to allow the lungs room to expand. The pillows, in fact, lean upon the patient, not the patient upon the pillows. It is impossible to give a rule for this, because it must vary with the figure of the patient. And tall patients suffer much more than short ones, because of the *drag* of the long limbs upon the waist. But the object is to support, with the pillows, the back *below* the breathing apparatus, to allow the shoulders room to fall back, and to support the head, without throwing it forward. The suffering of dying patients is immensely increased by neglect of these points. Any many an invalid, too weak to drag about his pillows himself, slips his book or anything at hand behind the lower part of his back to support it.

Helping the patient rest and sleep

We all take sleep for granted until we are deprived of it by pain or unhappiness – with its attendant tension – or the necessity for staying awake. Inability to rest and sleep adequately is both a cause and a consequence of disease. A patient is inherently subject to the stress caused by illness and confinement. But stress is a normal response to life, and only becomes pathological when tension is unrelieved by adequate periods of distraction or relaxation – or rest and sleep. Caregivers can do a great deal to increase the patient's disposition to benefit from a restful sleep. Everything that makes the day more pleasant for a patient, everything that increases the sense of well-being, everything that brings the patient at its close to feel that the day has been well spent increases the chances of natural sleep.

The removal of irritating stimuli, such as disagreeable sounds, odors or sights, will help to induce sleep; as will the relief of hunger. Even pleasurable excitement is to be avoided at bedtime. A massage at bedtime can be soporific, as are soft rhythmic sounds and rocking motions. Music can be sleep inducing. Well-chosen reading matter may be conducive to sleep because it diverts the mind from problems that are causing sleeplessness. Contact with another human being, or the evidence of another person's presence is comforting, even though the adult patient will rarely admit to loneliness or homesickness. The almost universal desire to be with family and friends as night falls needs to be acknowledged and satisfied as much as possible.

It is worth repeating here advice from Florence Nightingale on the importance of sleep, and the effects on a patient of having sleep disturbed.

> Never to allow a patient to be waked, intentionally or accidentally, is a sine qua non of all good nursing. If he is roused out of his first sleep, he is almost certain to have no more sleep. It is a curious but quite intelligible fact that, if a patient is waked after a few hours' instead of a few minutes' sleep, he is much more likely to sleep again. Because pain, like irritability of brain, perpetuates and intensifies itself. If you have gained a respite of either in

sleep you have gained more than the mere respite. Both the probability of recurrence and of the same intensity will be diminished; whereas both will be terribly increased by want of sleep. This is the reason why sleep is so all-important. This is the reason why a patient waked in the early part of his sleep loses not only his sleep, but his power to sleep.

Most individuals follow a simple pattern as preparation for sleep. For most patients this will include washing the face and hands, brushing the teeth, combing the hair, and seeing that the bedding is properly arranged and comfortable. Patients will most often prefer following this pattern themselves, but the caregiver may have to intervene and support the effort. The presence of the caregiver in the room at bedtime and the effect of the human touch goes a long way in overcoming tensions that build up after visitors leave and patients are alone with their thoughts.

Pressure sores

Pressure sores on the skin can arise in people of any age who are unable to reposition themselves in a bed or a chair. They frequently affect older individuals. Pressure sores usually develop below the waist, and usually over bony parts of the body such as the lower back, heels, elbows and hips. They may occur where pressure from a bed, chair, cast, splint or other hard object is in contact with the skin. They can be painful and even life-threatening.

Pressure sores occur when pressure on the skin reduces or cuts off the flow of blood bringing oxygen to the skin for a period of time, usually about 2–3 hours. The skin at the pressure point dies at the outer layer, the epidermis, and if left untended this can form an open sore or ulcer. Bacteria may enter through the broken skin to create infection. Most people do not develop pressure sores because they are always shifting position, without thinking about it, even when sleeping. People who are chronically ill, paralysed, comatose, very weak or restrained may be unable to move or to sense the discomfort or pain that normally signals the body to shift its position. Pressure sores can also arise through what is called 'traction,' when the skin sticks to something that exerts a pulling force upon it, like bed linens. Friction due to constant rubbing in an area of the skin is another cause of pressure sores. Skin moisture due to prolonged exposure to perspiration, urine or feces damages the skin making pressure sores more likely. Poor nutrition increases the risk of developing pressure sores and slows the process of them healing.

Pressure sores usually cause pain and itching, which may not be felt by patients whose senses are dulled by weakness or disease. There are four categories of pressure sores, from redness and inflammation of the skin (stage 1) to destruction of muscle, fat and bone (stage 4) at the point of pressure.

Preventing pressure sores

Pressure sores can be prevented by meticulous attention by the caregiver. Close, daily inspection of a bedridden or chair-bound patient's skin can detect early signs of pressure sore, usually redness or a discoloration of the skin. Any such sign is a signal that the patient needs to be repositioned and kept from lying or sitting on the discolored area until it returns to normal. Patients who cannot move them-selves should be repositioned at least every 2 hours, more often if possible. The skin needs to be kept clean and dry. Bony areas of the body, such as heels and elbows, can be protected with soft materials such as cotton or light wool. Special cushions, mattresses and other equipment have been developed to help prevent pressure sores. Caregivers should seek a recommendation from a physician or nurse on the appropriate equipment to use with the patient. None of these devices eliminate pressure sores completely, and there is simply no substitute for frequent repositioning of the patient.

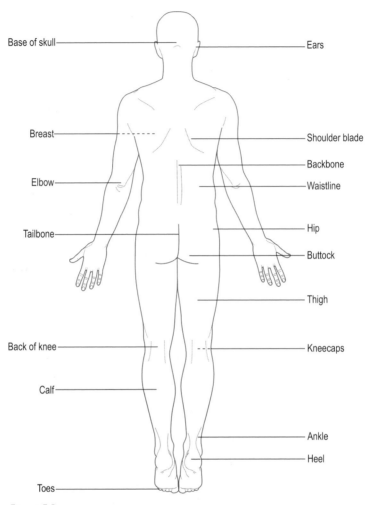

Figure 5.1

Locations where pressure sores can appear

The most vulnerable areas are the hips, heels, elbows and coccyx or tail bone. The sores can be caused by friction between the skin and the bed sheets. A bedsore can develop quickly, the damage varying from a change in skin color to wounds into the muscle or bone. The best prevention is to keep the skin dry and clean, with the patient's clothing worn loosely. The use of flannel or cotton sheets (100%) for bedding is best, because they absorb moisture. A patient who cannot leave the bed should be turned at least every 2 hours, to assume a new position. It is important to check the skin daily for the first signs of sores.

The caregiver should notify a physician or nurse at the first sign of bedsores. Meanwhile, measures can be taken, including:

- Removing pressure from the sore by changing the position of the patient.
- Wear disposable gloves when touching the patient to reduce the chance of infecting the sores.
- Avoid positions that put pressure on bony areas of the body.

Treating pressure sores

In the early stages, pressure sores usually heal by themselves once the pressure is removed. If the skin is broken, a physician or nurse needs to be consulted to recommend a treatment, usually a form of dressing.

Cleanliness

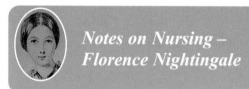

Notes on Nursing –
Florence Nightingale

Cleanliness of rooms and walls.

It cannot be necessary to tell a nurse that she should be clean, or that she should keep her patient clean, seeing that the greater part of nursing consists in preserving cleanliness. No ventilation can freshen a room or ward where the most scrupulous cleanliness is not observed. For a sick room, a carpet is perhaps the worst expedient which could by any possibility have been invented. If you must have a carpet, the only safety is to take it up two or three times a year, instead of once. A dirty carpet literally infects the room. And if you consider the enormous quantity of organic matter from the feet of people coming in, which must saturate it, this is by no means surprising.

Papers, plastered, oil-painted walls.

As for walls, the worst is the papered wall; the next worst is plaster. But the plaster can be redeemed by frequent lime-washing; the paper requires frequent renewing. A glazed paper gets rid of a good deal of the danger. But the ordinary bed-room paper is all that it ought not to be.

Air can be soiled just like water. If you blow into water you will soil it with the animal matter from your breath. So it is with air. Air is always soiled in a room where walls and carpets are saturated with animal exhalations. Want of cleanliness, then, in rooms and wards, which you have to guard against, may arise in three ways.

Dirty air from without.

Dirty air coming in from without, soiled by sewer emanations, the evaporation from dirty streets, smoke, bits of unburnt fuel, bits of straw, bits of horse dung.

Dirty air from within.

Dirty air coming from within, from dust, which you often displace, but never remove. And this recalls what ought to be a *sine qua non*. Have as few ledges in your room or ward as possible. And under no pretence have any ledge whatever out of sight. Dust accumulates there, and will never be wiped off. This is a certain way to soil the air.

Dirty air from carpet.

Dirty air coming from the carpet. Above all, take care of the carpets, that the animal dirt left there by the feet of visitors does not stay there. Floors, unless the grain is filled up and polished, are just as bad. The smell from the floor of a school-room or ward, when any moisture brings out the organic matter by which it is saturated, might alone be enough to warn us of the mischief that is going on.

Remedies.

Without cleanliness, you cannot have all the effect of ventilation; without ventilation, you can have no thorough cleanliness.

The well have a curious habit of forgetting that what is to them but a trifling inconvenience, to be patiently "put up" with, is to the sick a source of suffering, delaying recovery, if not actually hastening death. The well are scarcely ever more than eight hours, at most, in the same room. Some change they can always make, if only for a few minutes. Even during the supposed eight hours, they can change their posture or their position in the room. But the sick man who never leaves his bed, who cannot change by any movement of his own his air, or his light, or his warmth; who cannot obtain quiet, or get out of the smoke, or the smell, or the dust; he is really poisoned or depressed by what is to you the merest trifle.

"What can't be cured must be endured," is the very worst and most dangerous maxim for a nurse which ever was made. Patience and resignation in her are but other words for carelessness or indifference – contemptible, if in regard to herself; culpable, if in regard to her sick.

Personal cleanliness.

Poisoning by the skin.

In almost all diseases, the function of the skin is, more or less, disordered; and in many most important diseases nature relieves herself almost entirely by the skin. This is particularly the case with children. But the execretion, which comes from the skin, is left there, unless removed by washing or by the clothes. Every nurse should keep this fact constantly in mind, – for, if she allow her sick to remain unwashed, or their clothing to remain on them after being saturated with perspiration or other excretion, she is interfering injuriously with the natural processes of health just as effectually as if she were to give the patient a dose of slow poison by the mouth. Poisoning by the skin is no less certain than poisoning by the mouth – only it is slower in its operation.

Ventilation and skin-cleanliness equally essential.

The amount of relief and comfort experienced by the sick after the skin has been carefully washed and dried, is one of the commonest observations made at a sick bed. But it must not be forgotten that the comfort and relief so obtained are not all. They are, in fact, nothing more than a sign that the vital powers have been relieved by removing something that was oppressing them. The nurse, therefore, must never put off attending to the personal cleanliness of her patient under the plea that all that is to be gained is a little relief, which can be quite as well given later.

Just as it is necessary to renew the air round a sick person frequently, to carry off morbid effluvia from the lungs and skin, by maintaining free ventilation, so is it necessary to keep the pores of the skin free from all obstructing excretions. The object, both of ventilation and of skin-cleanliness, is pretty much the same, – to wit, removing noxious matter from the system as rapidly as possible.

Every nurse ought to be careful to wash her hands very frequently during the day. If her face too, so much the better.

Steaming and rubbing the skin.

One word as to cleanliness merely as cleanliness.

Compare the dirtiness of the water in which you have washed when it is cold without soap, cold with soap, hot with soap. You will find the first has hardly removed any dirt at all, the second a little more, the third a great deal more. But hold your hand over a cup of hot water for a minute or two, and then, by merely rubbing with the finger, you will bring off flakes of dirt or dirty skin. After a vapour bath you may peel your whole self clean in this way. What I mean is, that by simply washing or sponging with water you do not really clean your skin. Take a rough towel, dip one corner in very hot water, – if a little spirit be added to it it will be more effectual, – and then rub as if you were rubbing the towel into your skin with your fingers. The black flakes which will come off will convince you that you were not clean before, however much soap and water you have used. These flakes are what require removing. And you can really keep yourself cleaner with a tumbler of hot water and a rough towel and rubbing, than with a whole apparatus of bath and soap and sponge, without rubbing.

Helping the patient keep their body clean and well groomed

Cleanliness can be viewed from the two standpoints of its psychological and physiological values. Cleanliness and grooming are outward signs of a person's state of mind, and therefore closely related to a person's morale and state of mind. Thinking or seeing oneself as unkempt or unclean saps the spirit, especially for a patient suffering from an injury or illness. The role of the caregiver in cleanliness and grooming of a patient varies with each patient, and even over time with specific patients. However, it is generally best that patients be encouraged to assume as much responsibility as possible for their own cleanliness and grooming. This will necessarily change over time, and it is the job of the caregiver to assist in the transition towards diminishing or increasing levels of assistance.

The caregiver needs, in all cases, to ensure some basic conditions that favor cleanliness, and the independence of the patient in ensuring it is maintained. The patient should be provided with such facilities, equipment and assistance as needed to clean the skin, hair, nails, nose, mouth and teeth. Concepts of cleanliness vary, but patients should not have to lower their personal standards of cleanliness because they are sick.

Bathing and personal grooming • • •

A patient's condition may impose some changes on their grooming routine. For example, it may not be desirable to give a full bath daily – although most patients would enjoy it and benefit from it. The number of complete baths is, ideally, determined by the patient's physical needs and wishes. However, the bathing routine is also subject to instructions from a physician or nurse. In most cases, baths should be sufficiently frequent to give the appearance of cleanliness, to control body odors and to protect the skin from maceration and other forms of irritation.

Most patients in relatively good physical condition will prefer an immersion bath or shower, rather than a bed bath. Once again, the treating physician and nurse need to be consulted. In some cases the caregiver will need training or assistance in bathing a patient, or special equipment will need to be obtained, as recommended by the physician or nurse. There is a skill to making a bed bath both pleasurable and efficient, which the caregiver will need to acquire.

Personal grooming is also part of the psychological support provided for a patient. In most cases the caregiver can simply ensure everything is available for the patient to assume this task. Once again there are some simple guidelines. The hair should be thoroughly brushed at least once a day and kept well groomed according to the patient's standards. Washing the hair should be done according to the patient's wishes, but frequently enough to prevent disagreeable odors, and to keep the hair and scalp clean. A caregiver can give a shampoo to most bed patients without unduly tiring them and regardless of their position in bed. Once again, a nurse can provide guidance on the techniques the caregiver can use to do this properly, without discomfiting the patient.

Most men benefit from shaving daily. If able, they usually prefer to shave themselves. The caregiver should ensure all the proper materials are available. In some cases special

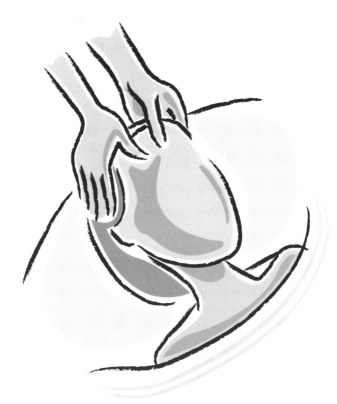

Figure 6.1

Personal grooming is important for the patient's psychological well-being as well as for hygiene

instructions from a health professional will need to be respected, such as the use of electric shavers rather than sharp instruments. The caregiver also needs to provide implements or help in keeping the nails and cuticles in good condition.

In some cases caregivers need to learn to clean the mouth and teeth of patients regardless of their state of consciousness and the position they must assume in bed. The teeth and gums need more thorough cleaning in illness than in health. The teeth should be brushed at least twice daily and preferably more often.

There are a few strategies that can help a caregiver to ensure the patient's attention to cleanliness and grooming. The caregiver can:

- Encourage the patient by ensuring comfort, warmth and privacy for bathing and showering.
- Make it possible for the patient to exercise preferences and personal choice in the use and replenishment of toiletries, cosmetics and clothing.
- Provide praise for good appearance.
- Be a role model for cleanliness and good grooming.

Helping the patient with elimination

A caregiver should be aware of the normal processes whereby the body eliminates various forms of waste, and should be able to detect changes in such processes, so they can be reported to a health professional. The patient will have 'normal' levels – for them – of, perspiring, urinating, menstruating and defecating. It is important for the caregiver to be able to monitor and judge these processes over time, as they are often important signs of changes in the condition of a patient, for better or for worse.

A caregiver should also be able to judge by odor or appearance when excretions are grossly abnormal. Certain abnormalities, such as a large bloody stool or bloody vomitus, call for immediate attention by the physician and possibly for emergency measures.

Eliminating, like eating, is closely tied up with the emotions. Stress is often associated with frequency in voiding, with diarrhea, or constipation. An anxious patient may want to void every hour and yet have no organic urinary disturbance. A depressed patient may go for days without having a bowel movement. Elimination of urine and excreta is a delicate matter, rendered more so in some cases by social or sexual taboos. Partly because urination, defecation, and menstruation are not topics of polite conversation, the average person is poorly informed about them, and therefore often finds difficulty in discussing them with health personnel, especially if they are of the opposite sex. All these social and physical considerations need to be considered in developing a plan of care that will enable the patient to function normally in this respect, while also preserving as much privacy and dignity as possible.

Female caregivers can encourage female patients to tell them what they may be embarrassed to tell men, and vice versa for male caregivers working with male patients who consult female health professionals. Privacy and physical comfort during defecation and voiding should be provided according to the demands of age and custom. In so far as it is possible, the physiological posture conducive to normal elimination should be encouraged. If a bed pan is required, the caregiver will need to obtain instruction on its use.

It is best to take the patient to the bathroom in a wheel-chair. Wheelchairs made into commodes can be substituted for the use of the bed pan if the patient can get out of bed. Such chairs are now made so that they fit over the toilet. In homes, ordinary armchairs may be converted into com-modes. Even for the seriously ill, the strain of emptying the rectum while in a semi-recumbent position may be far greater than that required to get out of bed and onto a commode for a bowel movement.

Care of the skin, provision for comfort, control of odors and prevention of chilling are problems with which the patient needs help whenever there is excessive sweating. This and excessively dry skin are conditions for which a physician or nurse may prescribe a treatment.

Since body excretions tend to have strong odors, the person unable to eliminate in private and to dispose of the excreta at once may suffer embarrassment and make others uncomfortable if this is not dealt with promptly and properly. It is up to the caregiver to reduce such problems to a minimum, if they cannot be completely overcome. The caregiver has also to be protected from contact with body discharges and to ensure that others are protected as well. Once again, this may require special methods or equipment, and advice should be sought from a health professional on what can be done. This will normally involve prompt removal of urine and excreta, and ensuring that receptacles are kept clean. In some cases, odors will also need to be dealt with by recourse to air conditioning, disinfectants and deodorants, although these are never substitutes for dealing with the cause of the odor, as much as possible.

Cleanliness and infections ● ● ●

Florence Nightingale came to understand the connection between cleanliness and the spread of infection, although the science of microbiology was yet to be developed when she began the practice of nursing. She learned from observation that dirt, foul air and unhygienic conditions spread disease; the measures she proposed to deal with these harmful conditions remain sound today in dealing with what we now know are various types of infection.

Most infections are caused by bacteria and viruses, tiny living creatures – called microorganisms – that are present everywhere in our environment. Many live on the skin, in the mouth and other parts of the human body. A healthy person lives in harmony with these parasites. The nature of a microorganism and the state of the person's natural defenses, the immune system, determine if a microorganism will remain benign or become a cause of disease. Infections are caused when viruses or bacteria begin to multiply in the body, overwhelming its defenses; or a state of balance may be achieved as the body fights back, producing a chronic infection; or the body, with or without medical treatment, may destroy the invading microorganisms. The main causes of infection are:

- **Bacteria:** these are microscopic single-celled organisms, such as *Streptococcus pyogenes*, the cause of 'strep' throat, and *Escherichia coli*, which results in urinary tract infection.

- **Viruses:** these are the smallest infectious organisms. They cannot reproduce on their own, but must invade a living cell to use the cell's machinery to reproduce. Examples include varicella zoster, which causes chickenpox and shingles, and rhinovirus, the cause of the common cold.

- **Fungi:** these are a type of plant. Yeasts, moulds and mushrooms are all types of fungi. Examples include *Candida albicans*, which causes vaginal yeast infection, and *Tinea pedis*, which results in athlete's foot.

- **Parasites:** these are organisms, such as worms or single-celled animals, that survive by living inside another, usually much larger organism or 'host'. Examples are *Enterobius vermicularis*, which is known as 'pinworm', and *Plasmodium falciparum*, the cause of malaria.

Physical barriers and the immune system usually defend the body against microorganisms. The physical barriers include the skin, mucous membranes, tears, earwax, mucus and stomach acid. The normal flow of urine washes out microorganisms that enter the urinary tract. The immune system uses white blood cells and antibodies to find and eliminate micro-organisms that get through the body's physical barriers.

What we call 'fever' is the increase of body temperature that occurs as a protective response to infection and injury. Temperature is considered elevated when it is higher than 100 degrees Fahrenheit (°F) as measured using an oral thermometer. Although 98.6°F is considered 'normal' temperature, body temperature varies throughout the day, being lowest in the morning and highest in the late afternoon – reaching up to 99.9°F.

The hypothalamus, in the human brain, controls body temperature. It raises the temperature of the body to a higher level by moving blood from the skin surface to the interior of the body, reducing heat loss through the skin. Shivering (experienced as chills) may be triggered to increase heat production through contraction of muscles. The body's measures to increase heat continue until blood reaches the hypothalamus at the new, higher temperature. The higher temperature is then maintained until the hypothalamus is reset to its normal level, with the body eliminating excess heat through sweating and the movement of blood to the skin.

Fever normally has an obvious cause, which is most often, but not always, an infection (e.g. influenza or pneumonia). A health professional can usually diagnose the cause of the fever by a physical examination and some simple tests. If fever persists over several days and has no obvious cause a more detailed investigation is required.

Preventing infection

There are procedures and practices the caregiver must learn to help prevent the spread of infection. They are especially important for regular activities, including:

- Serving meals and feeding the patient.
- Making beds.
- Assisting the patient with bathing and elimination.
- Handling dishes, bed pans and other implements used by the patient.
- Washing hands.

Human hands carry and transmit microorganisms, which means that frequent hand washing is an especially important means for preventing infection. Caregivers should develop the habit of washing hands frequently, using soap or special solutions. This is one of the single most important measures a caregiver can take to protect against infection. Contaminated hands represent a danger for the patient and the caregiver, as well as for family members and friends with whom the caregiver and the patient may have contact through the hands.

Hand washing can be done quickly and effectively by following some simple procedures. Hot water is best for washing hands, as it opens up the pores of the skin to remove microorganisms. Cuts, abrasions and skin lesions on the hands of a caregiver can be a source of infection. In such cases, in addition to washing hands, the caregiver should wear disposable gloves before attending to the patient.

There are ways of washing hands that are most effective. First, remove rings, watches, bracelets or other hand and wrist jewelry, as they frequently harbor microorganisms. It is advisable that caregivers who provide personal care not wear nail polish. The hands should be rubbed together vigorously, paying attention to the tips of the fingers, thumbs and areas between the fingers. Ensure that all surfaces are washed, including between the fingers and the back of the hand to 2 inches above the wrist, with a cleansing agent such as soap. Soap has detergent properties that effectively remove dirt, organic substances and transient flora from the skin. It is important to remember that some bacteria grow on bars of soap, especially if they are allowed to remain wet. Soap must be kept dry, or liquid soap can be used from a dispenser. In some cases, a health professional will propose use of an antiseptic preparation, which offers the benefit of killing or inhibiting the growth of resident microorganisms. Some antiseptic solutions used for hand washing continue to perform this function for several hours.

After lathering, the hands should be thoroughly rinsed, preferably under running water. If running water is not available, water can be poured from a container over the hands, or the hands can be rinsed in a bowl of water. This water has to be clean and should be changed after every use.

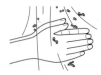
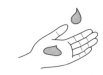
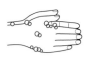

1. Wet hands and wrists under tepid running water.

2. Use a sufficient amount of soap or antiseptic as per manufacturer's instructions.

3. Lather soap and rub palms together.

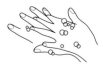

4. Rub in and between the fingers.

5. Rub back of each hand with palm of other hand.

6. Next, attend to the fingertips of each hand by rubbing them in opposite palm.

7. Then clean each thumb by clasping and rotating it in the opposite hand.

8. Rub each wrist clasped in opposite hand.

9. Rinse hands thoroughly, keeping hands lower than forearms.

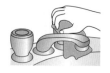

10. Blot hands dry with a paper towel, avoid rubbing harshly, as this will damage the skin.

11. Discard towel in an appropriate container without touching the bin or lid with hand.

12. Turn off water using a clean paper towel to avoid recontamination. **NB** This is not necessary if elbow or foot operated taps are available

Figure 6.2

Procedure for washing the hands – carefully!

The caregiver should keep nails short, as skin beneath the nails tends to accumulate high concentrations of bacteria. Any cuts or scratches on the hands should be cleaned and protected with an appropriate plaster or bandage, which should be changed often to ensure it does not become a source of infection.

Contamination of clothing

Microorganisms that can cause infection are everywhere. They can contaminate the clothing of caregivers unless preventive measures are respected. Caregivers should wear disposable gloves to handle dirty linen and should hold their gloved hands away from their clothing. It may be necessary to change clothing between tasks that can cause contamination, and those less likely to do so. Infected linen should be put into a bag, to be washed separately in very hot water.

Basic principles that should be respected by the caregiver to avoid infection include:

- Cuts and abrasions on the hands and arms of caregivers should be covered with waterproof plasters, which will provide a barrier against bacteria and viruses. The plasters should be changed frequently, since they may also become repositories of infection.

- Disposable latex or vinyl gloves should be worn in any situation where the hands may be contaminated with body fluids.

- Syringes and any other sharp objects must be disposed of carefully, in hard containers.

- Eating utensils should be washed immediately after meals. Disposable utensils are recommended in some cases.

The use of disposable gloves to handle food or to give personal care to patients can also help prevent the spread of infection. The caregiver should consult a health professional for advice.

Characteristics of local infection

If an infection develops it will be important for the caregiver to identify it as early as possible, so that the condition can be reported to a health professional for action.

The following are signs to watch for:

- Skin infections: these will usually produce inflammation that appears as a redness on the skin, sometimes accompanied by swelling and heat.

- Infection of the respiratory tract: signs usually include increased secretions, with symptoms such as coughing, sore throat and difficulty in breathing.

- Urinary tract infections: signs can include pain and increased frequency in passing urine. Symptoms can include a cloudy appearance, traces of blood in the urine and an abnormal 'fishy' smell.

- Gastrointestinal infections: signs can include abdominal pain, with symptoms such as nausea, vomiting, diarrhea and loss of appetite.

- Infections of the central nervous system: signs can include confusion and drowsiness, with symptoms such as a stiffness in the neck, headache and an increased sensitivity to light.

Bacterial infections

Antibiotics are generally effective against bacteria or fungi but they are ineffective against viruses. Antibiotics kill microorganisms or stop their reproduction so that they can be eliminated by the body's natural defenses. Each antibiotic works only against certain bacteria, and only a health professional can determine which will be most effective for a specific infection. Bacteria have the aptitude to change over time; some bacteria develop resistance to antibiotics. Ensuring that antibiotics are taken only when necessary helps limit this resistance.

Depending on the infection being treated, antibiotics may be given by injection or they can be taken orally. Antibiotics need to be taken until the infectious organism is eliminated. A course of antibiotics is rarely for less than 5 days. Discontinuing treatment too soon can result in a relapse of the infection or the development of antibiotic-resistant bacteria. A health professional – physician, nurse or pharmacist – can explain how the prescribed antibiotic should be administered to the patient. Some antibiotics must be taken on an empty stomach, whereas others need to be taken with food.

Fungal infections

Yeasts, moulds and mushrooms are all fungi. Some fungi reproduce by spreading microscopic spores in the air, from where they can be inhaled or come into contact with the body. This is why fungal infections usually begin in the lungs or on the skin. Most fungi that land on the skin or are inhaled do not cause infection, and they are rarely passed from one person to another. The normal balances in the body that keep fungi in check can be upset so that infections occur. For example, the bacteria normally present in the digestive tract and vagina limit the growth of certain fungi in those areas. Taking antibiotics can kill these helpful bacteria, allowing fungi to grow unchecked.

The risk factors for developing fungal infections include:

- Use of drugs that suppress the immune system, such as anticancer drugs (chemotherapy), corticosteroids and other immune-suppressant drugs.

- Diseases and conditions, including: AIDS; kidney failure; diabetes; lung disease, such as emphysema; Hodgkin's disease or other lymphomas; leukemia; extensive burns; and organ transplantation.

Medications can be used against fungal infections, but the structure and chemical composition of fungi make them difficult to kill. Antifungal medications may be applied directly to a fungal infection on the skin. Some may be taken orally or injected to treat more serious infections. Several months of treatment are often needed.

Viral infections

Viruses are the cause of human ailments ranging from the common cold to rabies, hepatitis and smallpox. The human immunodeficiency virus (HIV) infection is caused by two viruses HIV-1 and HIV-2. A virus is a microorganism that is smaller than a fungus or a bacterium, and which needs to invade a living cell in order to reproduce. The virus attaches to and enters a cell, and releases the DNA or RNA that contains the information for its replication. The host cell follows these instructions to reproduce the virus. The infected cell usually dies, but not before releasing other viruses that go on to infect other cells. In some cases host cells are not killed but lose control over normal cell division so that they become cancerous. Some viruses that do not kill infected cells leave their genetic material in the cell where it remains dormant. This is referred to as a 'latent infection'. The dormant material may be able to grow again after a period of time and cause disease. Individual viruses usually infect only one type of cell. For example, cold viruses infect only cells of the upper respiratory tract. Viruses enter the body in a number of ways; for example, they may be inhaled, swallowed or transmitted through the bites of mosquitoes and other insects.

The body defends itself against viruses with physical barriers, such as the skin, and by activating defenses in the immune system. White blood cells attack and destroy the virus or the cells it has infected. These white blood cells, some of which are called 'lymphocytes', 'remember' the characteristics of the invading virus, enabling them to respond more quickly and effectively to future invasions by the same virus. This is the mechanism we know as 'immunity', which is also the basis for the effectiveness of vaccines. Infected cells can also produce substances called 'interferons', which increase the resistance to infection of non-infected cells.

Antiviral drugs have been developed to fight viruses, mainly by interfering with their replication. The nature of viruses, their size and their method of replication make it difficult to attack them using drugs. Bacteria and fungi, for example, are much more susceptible to this form of attack because they are larger and have many metabolic functions against which drugs can be directed. Antiviral drugs are difficult to develop, and some can be toxic to human cells. Viruses are also able to develop resistance to antiviral drugs. Antibiotics are not effective against viral infections, although they may be used for a patient who has both a viral and a bacterial infection.

Vaccines

Vaccines have been developed to help the body's cells fight against infection by viruses. Vaccines contain inactivated (killed) versions of a specific virus or pieces of that virus. The influenza vaccine, for example, protects against three different strains of the influenza virus. Different vaccines may be given every year to keep up with the changes in the influenza virus. Experts assess which strain of virus will attack in the next year based on identifying the strain of the virus that predominated in the current flu season and the strain of the virus causing influenza in other parts of the world.

Vaccination against influenza is particularly important for people who are most susceptible to becoming very ill, including the young, those over 50 years of age and anyone with a chronic illness such as diabetes, lung disease or heart disease. The caregiver must consult a health professional about the need or desirability of vaccination for the person being cared for.

7

Chattering Hopes and Advices

Notes on Nursing – Florence Nightingale

Chattering hopes the bane of the sick.

"Chattering Hopes" may seem an odd heading. But I really believe there is scarcely a greater worry which invalids have to endure than the incurable hopes of their friends. There is no one practice against which I can speak more strongly from actual personal experience, wide and long, of its effects during sickness observed both upon others and upon myself. I would appeal most seriously to all friends, visitors, and attendants of the sick to leave off this practice of attempting to "cheer" the sick by making light of their danger and by exaggerating their probabilities of recovery.

Far more now than formerly does the medical attendant tell the truth to the sick who are really desirous to hear it about their own state.

How intense is the folly, then, to say the least of it, of the friend, be he even a medical man, who thinks that his opinion, given after a cursory observation, will weigh with the patient, against the opinion of the medical attendant, given, perhaps, after years of observation, after using every help to diagnosis afforded by the stethoscope, the examination of pulse, tongue, &c.; and certainly after much more observation than the friend can possibly have had.

Patient does not want to talk of himself.

The fact is, that the patient is not "cheered" at all by these well-meaning, most tiresome friends. On the contrary, he is depressed and wearied. If, on the one hand, he exerts himself to tell each successive member of this too numerous conspiracy, whose name is legion, why he does not think as they do, – in what respect he is worse, – what symptoms exist that they know nothing of, – he is fatigued instead of "cheered," and his attention is fixed upon himself. In general, patients who are really ill, do not want to talk about themselves. Hypochondriacs do, but again I say we are not on the subject of hypochondriacs.

Absurd consolations put forth for the benefit of the sick.

If, on the other hand, and which is much more frequently the case, the patient says nothing, but the Shakespearian "Oh!" "Ah!" "Go to!" and "In good sooth!" in order to escape from the conversation about himself the sooner, he is depressed by want of sympathy. He feels isolated in the midst of friends. He feels what a convenience it would be, if there were any single person to whom he could speak simply and openly, without pulling the string upon himself of this shower-bath of silly hopes and encouragements; to whom he could express his wishes and directions without that person persisting in saying, "I hope that it will please God yet to give you twenty years," or, "You have a long life of activity before you." How often we see at the end of biographies of cases recorded in medical papers, "after a long illness A. died rather suddenly," or, "unexpectedly both to himself and to others." "Unexpectedly" to others, perhaps, who did not see, because they did not look; but by no means "unexpectedly to himself," as I feel entitled to believe, both from the internal evidence in such stories, and from watching similar cases; there was every reason to expect that A. would die, and he knew it; but he found it useless to insist upon his own knowledge to his friends.

In these remarks I am alluding neither to acute cases which terminate rapidly nor to "nervous" cases.

By the first much interest in their own danger is very rarely felt. In writings of fiction, whether novels or biographies, these death-beds are generally depicted as almost seraphic in lucidity of intelligence. Sadly large has been my experience in death-beds, and I can only say that I have seldom or never seen such. Indifference, excepting with regard to bodily suffering, or to some duty the dying man desires to perform, is the far more usual state.

The "nervous case," on the other hand, delights in figuring to himself and others a fictitious danger.

But the long chronic case, who knows too well himself, and who has been told by his physician that he will never enter active life again, who feels that every month he has to give up something he could do the month before – oh! spare such sufferers your chattering hopes. You do not know how you worry and weary them. Such real sufferers cannot bear to talk of themselves, still less to hope for what they cannot at all expect.

So also as to all the advice showered so profusely upon such sick, to leave off some occupation, to try some other doctor, some other house, climate, pill, powder, or specific; I say nothing of the inconsistency – for these advisers are sure to be the same persons who exhorted the sick man not to believe his own doctor's prognostics, because "doctors are always mistaken," but to believe some other doctor, because "this doctor is always right." Sure also are these advisers to be the persons to bring

the sick man fresh occupation, while exhorting him to leave
his own.

Wonderful presumption of the advisers to the sick.

Wonderful is the face with which friends, lay and medical, will
come in and worry the patient with recommendations to do
something or other, having just as little knowledge as to its being
feasible, or even safe for him, as if they were to recommend a
man to take exercise, not knowing he had broken his leg. What
would the friend say, if *he* were the medical attendant, and if
the patient, because some *other* friend had come in, because
somebody, anybody, nobody, had recommended something,
anything, nothing, were to disregard his orders, and take that
other body's recommendation? But people never think of this.

To me these commonplaces, leaving their smear upon the
cheerful, single-hearted, constant devotion to duty, which is so
often seen in the decline of such sufferers, recall the slimy trail left
by the snail on the sunny southern garden-wall loaded with fruit.

Mockery of the advice given to the sick.

No mockery in the world is so hollow as the advice showered
upon the sick. It is of no use for the sick to say anything, for
what the adviser wants is, *not* to know the truth about the state
of the patient, but to turn whatever the sick may say to the
support of his own argument, set forth, it must be repeated,
without any inquiry whatever into the patient's real condition."

To nurses I say – these are the visitors who do your patient harm.

How little the real sufferings of illness are known or understood.
How little does any one in good health fancy him or even
*her*self into the life of a sick person.

Means of giving pleasure to the sick.

Do, you who are about the sick or who visit the sick, try and give them pleasure, remember to tell them what will do so. How often in such visits the sick person has to do the whole conversation, exerting his own imagination and memory, while you would take the visitor, absorbed in his own anxieties, making no effort of memory or imagination, for the sick person. "Oh! my dear, I have so much to think of, I really quite forgot to tell him that; besides, I thought he would know it," says the visitor to another friend. How could "he know it?" Depend upon it, the people who say this are really those who have little "to think of." There are many burthened with business who always manage to keep a pigeon-hole in their minds, full of things to tell the "invalid."

I do not say, don't tell him your anxieties – I believe it is good for him and good for you too; but if you tell him what is anxious, surely you can remember to tell him what is pleasant too.

A sick person does so enjoy hearing good news: – for instance, of a love and courtship, while in progress to a good ending. If you tell him only when the marriage takes place, he loses half the pleasure, which God knows he has little enough of; and ten to one but you have told him of some love-making with a bad ending.

A sick person also intensely enjoys hearing of any *material* good, any positive, or practical success of the right. He has so much of books and fiction, of principles, and precepts, and theories; do, instead of advising him with advice he has heard at least fifty times before, tell him of one benevolent act which has really succeeded practically, – it is like a day's health to him.

You have no idea what the craving of sick with undiminished power of thinking, but little power of doing, is to hear of good practical action, when they can no longer partake in it.

Do observe these things with the sick. Do remember how their life is to them disappointed and incomplete. You see them lying there with miserable disappointments, from which they can have no escape but death, and you can't remember to tell them of what would give them so much pleasure, or at least an hour's variety.

They don't want you to be lachrymose and whining with them, they like you to be fresh and active and interested, but they cannot bear absence of mind, and they are so tired of the advice and preaching they receive from everybody, no matter whom it is, they see.

There is no better society than babies and sick people for one another. Of course you must manage this so that neither shall suffer from it, which is perfectly possible. If you think the "air of the sick room" bad for the baby, why it is bad for the invalid too, and, therefore, you will of course correct it for both. It freshens up a sick person's whole mental atmosphere to see "the baby." And a very young child, if unspoiled, will generally adapt itself wonderfully to the ways of a sick person, if the time they spend together is not too long.

If you knew how unreasonably sick people suffer from reasonable causes of distress, you would take more pains about all these things. An infant laid upon the sick bed will do the sick person, thus suffering, more good than all your logic. A piece of good news will do the same. Perhaps you are afraid of "disturbing" him. You say there is no comfort for his present cause of affliction. It is perfectly reasonable. The distinction is this, if he is obliged to act, do not "disturb" him with another subject of thought just yet; help him to do what he wants to do; but, if he has done this, or if nothing can be done, then "disturb" him by all means. You will relieve, more effectually, unreasonable suffering from reasonable causes by telling him "the news," showing him "the baby," or giving him something new to think of or to look at than by all the logic in the world.

It has been very justly said that the sick are like children in this, that there is no *proportion* in events to them. Now it is your business as their visitor to restore this right proportion for them – to show them what the rest of the world is doing. How can they find it out otherwise? You will find them far more open to conviction than children in this. And you will find that their unreasonable intensity of suffering from unkindness, from want of sympathy, &c., will disappear with their freshened interest in the big world's events. But then you must be able to give them real interests, not gossip.

Fundamental needs

A caregiver who spends most days with a patient, taking meals, discussing every-day events, sharing opinions and concerns, necessarily becomes one of the people most sensitive to the patient's thoughts, fears and general morale. Understanding a patient's mentality is important for the caregiver in terms of the quality of the care provided, and it is important to the patient as a stimulus to recovery. Providing care at home is a personal commitment, imbued with complicated emotions of love, worry and even frustration.

Caregivers are most likely to understand the patient's behavior if they share their interpretation of it, which requires developing the talent for communicating with the patient. For example, the caregiver may say 'You look to me as if you are worried' or 'in pain' or 'angry.' Very often if the caregiver uses such an approach, repeating what they believe are the patient's thoughts, the patient can be encouraged to unburden themselves of fears they scarcely realized they had. The caregiver might say, for example, 'Are you telling me that you are more afraid to be made unconscious by the anaesthetic than to have the operation?' In answering, patients may identify the fears they are reluctant to accept or to discuss with others. Having identified such fears, both the patient and the caregiver are in a position to share the information with a physician or nurse, who will assist both in coping with them. Of course, the caregiver must always be attentive to the need for confidentiality in matters that are discussed with the patient. These should not be shared with others without the knowledge and consent of the patient. There are, however, situations where caregivers will need to exercise judgement about what information to share. In some cases it will be invaluable that the caregiver makes a physician or nurse aware of information that has been confided by the patient.

'A constructive relationship' in the therapeutic setting is so essential that the caregiver must make an effort to help the patient communicate hopes, frustrations, fear, anger, love, and other emotions. The caregiver's self-awareness (the ability to recognize one's own emotional problems, to asses one's qualities, talents and also liabilities) affects the capacity for fulfilling this demanding function. The injunction of the ancient Greeks to 'Know thyself' and Shakespeare's advice: 'To thine own self be true' are classic expressions of this human faculty; the understanding that self-knowledge and self-respect are fundamental to the understanding of, and respect for, others. The ways in which this respect manifests itself may be banal. They can include simple aspects of daily life which most of us take for granted. However, the caregiver comes to understand that for someone with limited physical ability, confined to a sick bed or room, these simple tasks become the focus of whatever pleasure and encouragement the patient can derive from each day that goes by.

Helping the patient with selection of clothing, with dressing and undressing ● ● ●

Providing care for a patient may include helping make a suitable choice of clothing, both in terms of warmth, protection or simply to favor a pleasing appearance. In this respect, a caregiver should consider a patient's choice of clothing and the desire to 'look good' as an extension of the personality. A patient will select garments that express preferences and individuality. It is especially important for a patient who is not able to dress alone that they be consulted in the choice of clothing. A dress or shirt that the patient finds plain or uncongenial may considerably depress or disturb them. Conversely, dressing well, according to a patient's tastes, can enhance self-respect if the wearer believes it enhances his appearance and status. Dressing is one of the functions we all see as commonplace. It is when we lose the freedom to choose what we will wear, how we will appear to others, that we become more susceptible to the feelings of helplessness and dejection that illness can induce.

Day and night are marked for most people by a change of clothing, as are regular activities such as going out, taking meals, etc. This normal cycle is broken when a patient spends most of every day in garments designed for rest and sleep; often contributing to the disorientation and sense of hopelessness seen during illness. With this in mind, the caregiver should work with the patient to reduce to a minimum the interruption of normal habits of dressing. Illness may at times constrain choice and variety of dress, but this should not become a pretext for ignoring the importance that dressing well, exercising a choice of garments, etc. plays in the psychological state of a patient, and therefore in the process of healing and recovery.

For the sick and disabled, the caregiver may need to supply the physical support needed for dressing and undressing. This support needs to be provided thoughtfully, remembering always to let the patient take on as much of the effort as possible; remembering also that dressing and undressing are highly personal matters that most of us prefer to do in private. The caregiver needs to be considerate and sensitive to the patient's feelings in this respect, while still ensuring safety is not compromised by letting the patient take on more than can be handled.

Helping the patient communicate with others to express needs and feelings • • •

Anyone who has worked with ailing patients is quickly reminded of the basic truth that the human psyche (mind) and the soma (body) are interdependent and inseparable. Every emotion we experience has a physical expression, and this physical change is in turn interpreted as emotion. We interpret a quickened heart beat and respiratory rate, accompanied by a flushed appearance, as the effects of emotion. In this case these physical manifestations are seen as symptoms of 'excitement.' The opposite appearance, such as stooped posture, weak voice and an immobile face, represent a state of sadness or depression.

If we accept that emotions are inevitably associated with physical change, it is not hard to embrace the concept that some of these reactions may be constructive or helpful to the patient, while others are destructive. All of us attempt in our own way to express our thoughts, emotions and desires, and we have an equal desire to understand and empathize with others through a process of communication, verbally and through other means. Someone who is ill and dependent upon others for care retains nonetheless a desire to be helpful in contributing to the happiness of others.

It may seem presumptuous to suggest that caregivers should assist the persons they care for with any function so complex, so individual, and so bound up with the total personality as communication. The simple reality is that the caregiver is inescapably, among other things, an interpreter for the patient vis à vis the world outside the confines of an illness. The caregiver can often facilitate communication with family and friends, sometimes by providing information on the condition and status of the patient that the latter may not wish to broach alone. This aspect of a caregiver's role contributes to fostering happy relationships for the patient, and thus promotes mental and physical well-being.

A more difficult role for the caregiver is that of helping patients to understand themselves, to alter conditions that are making them sick and to accept those that cannot be changed. This is a function that the caregiver shares with relatives, friends and other caregivers. The self-awareness a caregiver needs to develop includes understanding the need to be inclusive in this important role, and to defer when necessary to others who are closer to the patient or better equipped professionally to deal with a problem.

There is no question that separation from family and friends and the fear of altered relationships are responsible for much of the suffering attendant upon sickness. Likewise, family and friends suffer when the threat of death makes patients concentrate all their energy on recovery, for in such cases patients may appear totally indifferent to them. The more understanding the caregiver, the more the care-giver invites the confidence of the patient and his family, the better he or she is able to help the patient overcome the psychological hazards of illness. A caregiver who accepts the interpreter–communicator role welcomes opportunities to be with their patients and to meet their family, friends and associates, to listen and to talk with them. A caregiver who assumes this role thoughtfully is invaluable to a patient in many respects that go beyond simple, physical care. A care-giver can be instrumental in fostering relationships for the patient; for example, by getting a needed relative, friend or religious adviser to visit the patient or to raise with them an issue the patient wishes to discuss. The nature of the relationship between a caregiver and patient is such that it includes a responsibility to help the patient maintain satisfying ways of expressing their needs, interests and desires.

Helping the patient with work, or productive occupation ● ● ●

A normal day for most people includes doing something that is seen as useful. The product of the activity may be a material object that has been fashioned with the hands, or some knowledge acquired through the various senses.

In most cultures there is an expectation that adults will produce something useful, and when they do not conform to this practice society shows its disapproval. This becomes an innate measure that individuals apply to themselves. It is one reason why sickness loses some of its terror for most people if they can continue to do something they and others will judge to be useful work. If people are productive mentally, and within their limits physically, they can spend years confined to bed and live to a ripe old age. Florence Nightingale, for example, spent half her life confined to her room, and usually to her bed, but when all her letters to people around the world are considered as her 'work' she may prove to have had the largest correspondence ever known. Throughout her years of confinement she wrote with advice and recommendations to Queen Victoria, to government ministers and officials, to journalists, and to friends and family. To this we can add the large body of personal 'Notes' she wrote, many of which were instrumental in forming public opinion and reforming public policy on matters of public hygiene, hospitals and nursing. The work that she accomplished as an 'invalid' is as remarkable as that performed during her so-called 'active' years.

The caregiver should watch for signs of interest in work, and seek to introduce opportunities for patients to do something that gives them a sense of achievement. This can be as simple as learning, or taking up again, a favorite handicraft or artistic pursuit such as painting and drawing. It can also be an activity from the patient's former working life, and as such can furnish a gentle transition back from illness to regular work. The essential quality for whatever activities are pursued is that they should be enjoyable and satisfying for the patient. This aspect of caregiving is also related to the importance of helping the patient to retain and to regain independence.

The caregiver who helps a patient plan the day should encourage any 'work' interests they have, and try to ensure that the environment is conducive to this productive activity. As in all aspects of care, judgement in the interpretation of the patient's needs and energies is essential. Nature endows all organisms with the will to survive, and when a living entity is threatened all energies are invested in survival. It is unrealistic to expect the critically ill person to be concerned with much else. There is no doubt, however, that interest in what they still hoped to accomplish has wrought what appears to be 'miracles' of healing in human beings.

Helping the patient with recreational activities • • •

Recreation, or play, in contrast to work, is activity undertaken for the enjoyment of it rather than for the sake of the product. Most people analyzing their average day will find some part of it spent in: listening to music; reading for pleasure, rather than edification; playing a game; watching television or a video; going to a theatre, a museum or a 'party;' or riding, swimming, walking, driving, dancing or exercising in some enjoyable fashion. Even shopping can be a form of recreation.

Too often sickness deprives its victim of opportunities for variety and refreshment, for relief, or recreation. Sometimes this deprivation is necessary; much more often it results from the failure of well persons to provide conditions that make recreation for the sick possible. The patient may be thoughtlessly and needlessly confined to one room; too often put into clothing associated in his mind with sleep, or inactivity, and deprived of every pleasurable resource.

In making any plan for basic care, a caregiver should consider what hours of the patient's day might be set aside for recreation, what are the patient's recreational interests and what facilities are available to pursue this activity. The selection of specific activities depends upon the patient's gender, age, intelligence, experience and tastes; and upon the condition, or the severity of the illness; upon the patient's enjoyment of exercise and of the arts; and, of course, upon the resources for games and companionship. Much more depends upon the imagination and the talents of the caregiver, of the patients and their associates, than upon any physical resources.

To begin with, few patients need to be limited to one room. At home it is rarely necessary to keep the sick person confined. But, even during confinement, the arrangement and furnishing of the room can be changed occasionally to provide variety and to introduce elements of aesthetic enjoyment into the occupant's life.

Reading materials are available in most situations. Daily and weekly papers can help to keep the sick feeling that they are 'in the stream of life.' Libraries on wheels and other such resources can provide a wide variety of recreational, as well as instructive, books, pamphlets and periodicals. These and other outlets are also sources of films, plays and television programs on DVDs and other electronic media. Patients who are too sick or incapacitated to read to themselves enjoy being read to or listening to 'talking books.' Music and the theatre are increasingly available to the sick and handicapped because of the widespread availability of radio, television, and home video players.

Even shopping, either in person or on the Internet, can be a great source of recreation and pleasure. There is no way of measuring the possible benefits to a sick person from surprising a spouse with a birthday present, or the lift it gives a disabled older person to watch a grandchild's pleasure as he opens a gift.

Observation of the Sick

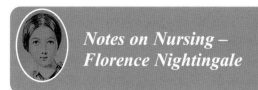

Notes on Nursing – Florence Nightingale

What is the use of the question, Is he better?

There is no more silly or universal question scarcely asked than this, "Is he better?" What you want are facts, not opinion – for who can have any opinion of any value as to whether the patient is better or worse, excepting the constant medical attendant, or the really observing nurse?

The most important practical lesson that can be given to Nurses is to teach them what to observe – how to observe – what symptoms indicate improvement – what the reverse – which are of importance – which are of none – which are the evidence of neglect – and of what kind of neglect.

The vagueness and looseness of the information one receives in answer to that much abused question, "Is he better?" would be ludicrous, if it were not painful.

I can record but a very few specimens of the answers which I have heard made by friends and Nurses, and accepted by physicians and surgeons at the very bed-side of the patient, who could have contradicted every word, but did not – sometimes from amiability, often from shyness, oftenest from languor!

"How often have the bowels acted, nurse?" "Once, sir." This generally means that the utensil has been emptied once, it having been used perhaps seven or eight times.

"Do you think the patient is much weaker than he was six weeks ago?" "Oh no, sir; you know it is very long since he has been up and dressed, and he can get across the room now." This means that the nurse has not observed that whereas six weeks ago he sat up and occupied himself in bed, he now lies still doing nothing; that, although he can "get across the room," he cannot stand for five seconds.

Another patient who is eating well, recovering steadily, although slowly, from fever, but cannot walk or stand, is represented to the physician as making no progress at all.

Leading questions useless or misleading.

Questions, too, as asked now (but too generally) of or about patients, would obtain no information at all about them, even if the person asked of had every information to give. The question is generally a leading question; and it is singular that people never think what must be the answer to this question before they ask it: for instance, "Has he had a good night?" Now, one patient will think he has a bad night if he has not slept ten hours without waking. Another does not think he has a bad night if he has had intervals of dosing occasionally. The same answer has actually been given as regarded two patients – one who had been entirely sleepless for five times twenty-four hours, and died of it, and another who had not slept the sleep of a regular night, without waking. Why cannot the question be asked, How many hours' sleep has — had? and at what hours of the night?

How few there are who, by five or six pointed questions, can elicit the whole case, and get accurately to know and to be able to report where the patient is.

Means of obtaining inaccurate information.

I knew a very clever physician, of large dispensary and hospital practice, who invariably began his examination of each patient with "Put your finger where you be bad." That man would never waste his time with collecting inaccurate information from nurse or patient. Leading questions always collect inaccurate information.

As to food patient takes or does not take.

It is useless to go through all the particulars, besides sleep, in which people have a peculiar talent for gleaning inaccurate information. As to food, for instance, I often think that most common question, How is your appetite? can only be put because the questioner believes the questioned has really nothing the matter with him, which is very often the case. But where there is, the remark holds good which has been made about sleep. The *same* answer will often be made as regards a patient who cannot take two ounces of solid food per diem, and a patient who does not enjoy five meals a day as much as usual.

Again, the question, How is your appetite? is often put when How is your digestion? is the question meant. No doubt the two things depend on one another. But they are quite different. Many a patient can eat, if you can only "tempt his appetite." The fault lies in your not having got him the thing that he fancies. But many another patient does not care between grapes and turnips – everything is equally distasteful to him. He would try to eat anything which would do him good; but every thing "makes him worse." The fault here generally lies in the cooking. It is not his "appetite" which requires "tempting," it is his digestion which requires sparing. And good sick cookery will save the digestion half its work.

There may be four different causes, any one of which will produce the same result, viz., the patient slowly starving to death from want of nutrition:

Defect in cooking;

Defect in choice of diet;

Defect in choice of hours for taking diet;

Defect of appetite in patient.

Yet all these are generally comprehended in the one sweeping assertion that the patient has "no appetite."

Surely many lives might be saved by drawing a closer distinction; for the remedies are as diverse as the causes. The remedy for the first is to cook better; for the second, to choose other articles of diet; for the third, to watch for the hours when the patient is in want of food; for the fourth, to show him what he likes, and sometimes unexpectedly. But no one of these remedies will do for any other of the defects not corresponding with it.

I cannot too often repeat that patients are generally either too languid to observe these things, or too shy to speak about them; nor is it well that they should be made to observe them, it fixes their attention upon themselves.

Again, I say, what *is* the nurse or friend there for except to take note of these things, instead of the patient doing so?

For it may safely be said, not that the habit of ready and correct observation will by itself make us useful Nurses, but that without it we shall be useless with all our devotion.

I have known a nurse in charge of a set of wards, who not only carried in her head all the little varieties in the diets which each patient was allowed to fix for himself, but also exactly what each patient had taken during each day. I have known another nurse in charge of one single patient, who took away his meals day after day all but untouched, and never knew it.

If you find it helps you to note down such things on a bit of paper, in pencil, by all means do so. I think it more often lames than strengthens the memory and observation. But if you cannot get the habit of observation one way or other, you had better give up the being a nurse, for it is not your calling, however kind and anxious you may be.

Surely you can learn at least to judge with the eye how much an oz. of solid food is, how much an oz. of liquid. You will find this helps your observation and memory very much, you will then say to yourself, "A. took about an oz. of his meat today;" "B. took three times in 24 hours about ¼ pint of beef tea;" instead of saying "B. has taken nothing all day," or "I gave A. his dinner as usual."

Superstition the fruit of bad observation.

Almost all superstitions are owing to bad observation, to the *post hoc, ergo propter hoc*; and bad observers are almost all superstitious. Farmers used to attribute disease among cattle to witchcraft; weddings have been attributed to seeing one magpie, deaths to seeing three; and I have heard the most highly educated now-a-days draw consequences for the sick closely resembling these.

Physiogonomy of disease little shewn by the face.

Another remark: although there is unquestionably a physiognomy of disease as well as of health; of all parts of the body, the face is perhaps the one which tells the least to the common observer or the casual visitor. Because, of all parts of the body, it is the one most exposed to other influences, besides health. And people never, or scarcely ever, observe enough to know how to distinguish between the effect of exposure, of robust health, of a tender skin, of a tendency to congestion, of suffusion, flushing, or many other things. Again, the face is often the last to shew emaciation. I should say that the hand was a much surer test than the face, both as to flesh, colour, circulation, &c., &c. It is true that there are *some* diseases which are only betrayed at all by something in the face, *e.g.*, the eye or the tongue, as great irritability of brain by the appearance of the pupil of the eye. But we are talking of casual, not minute, observation. And few minute observers will hesitate to say that far more untruth than truth is conveyed by the oft repeated words, He *looks* well, or ill, or better or worse.

I have known patients dying of sheer pain, exhaustion, and want of sleep, from one of the most lingering and painful diseases known, preserve, till within a few days of death, not only the healthy colour of the cheek, but the mottled appearance of a robust child. And scores of times have I heard these unfortunate creatures assailed with, "I am glad to see you looking so well." "I see no reason why you should not live till ninety years of age." "Why don't you take a little more exercise and amusement," with all the other commonplaces with which we are so familiar.

There is, unquestionably, a physiognomy of disease. Let the nurse learn it.

The experienced nurse can always tell that a person has taken a narcotic the night before by the patchiness of the colour about the face, when the re-action of depression has set in; that very colour which the inexperienced will point to as a proof of health.

There is, again, a faintness, which does not betray itself by the colour at all, or in which the patient becomes brown instead of white. There is a faintness of another kind which, it is true, can always be seen by the paleness. But the nurse seldom distinguishes. Yet these two faintnesses are perfectly distinguishable, by the mere countenance of the patient.

Peculiarities of patients.

Again, the nurse must distinguish between the idiosyncracies of patients. One likes to suffer out all his suffering alone, to be as little looked after as possible. Another likes to be perpetually made much of and pitied, and to have someone always by him. Both these peculiarities might be observed and indulged much more than they are. For quite as often does it happen that a busy attendance is forced upon the first patient, who wishes for nothing but to be "let alone," as that the second is left to think himself neglected. Nurse must observe for herself increase of patient's weakness, patient will not tell her.

Again, I think that few things press so heavily on one suffering from long and incurable illness, as the necessity of recording in words from time to time, for the information of the nurse, who will not otherwise see, that he cannot do this or that, which he could do a month or a year ago. What is a nurse there for if she cannot observe these things for herself?

Let people who have to observe sickness and death look back and try to register in their observation the appearances which have preceded relapse, attack, or death, and not assert that there were none, or that there were not the right ones.

Observation of general conditions.

A want of the habit of observing conditions and an inveterate habit of taking averages are each of them often equally misleading.

What observation is for.

In dwelling upon the vital importance of sound observation, it must never be lost sight of what observation is for. It is not for the sake of piling up miscellaneous information or curious facts, but for the sake of saving life and increasing health and comfort. The caution may seem useless, but it is quite surprising how many men (some women do it too), practically behave as if the scientific end were the only one in view, or as if the sick body were but a reservoir for stowing medicines into, and the surgical disease only a curious case the sufferer has made for the attendant's special information. This is really no exaggeration. You think, if you suspected your patient was being poisoned, say, by a copper kettle, you would instantly, as you ought, cut off all possible connection between him and the suspected source of injury, without regard to the fact that a curious mine of observation is thereby lost. But it is not everybody who does so, and it has actually been made a question of medical ethics, what should the medical man do if he suspected poisoning? The answer seems a very simple one, – insist on a confidential nurse being placed with the patient, or give up the case.

What a confidential nurse should be.

And remember every nurse should be one who is to be depended upon, in other words, capable of being a "confidential" nurse. She does not know how soon she may find herself placed in such a situation; she must be no gossip, no vain talker; she should never answer questions about her sick except to those who have a right to ask them; she must, I need not say, be strictly sober and honest; but more than this, she must be a religious and devoted woman; she must have a respect for her own calling, because God's precious gift of life is often literally placed in her hands; she must be a sound, and close, and quick observer; and she must be a woman of delicate and decent feeling.

Observation of the patient

The physician or nurse who is treating a patient sees them at most a few hours in any single week. It remains as important today as it was in Florence Nightingale's time for the regular caregiver to be attentive to the condition of the patient. No one is better placed to notice small variations or changes in mood, in appetite or in some physical aspect of the patient. The caregiver will not understand the significance of everything observed, but noting down any observations and conveying them to the physician or nurse on a regular basis is an invaluable part of care that only the caregiver can provide.

The caregiver who assumes this role will hone the natural sense of observation, and will learn to be attentive to specific signs. Any such observations should be written down as a matter of daily routine. In addition to serving as an aid to memory for discussions about the patient with health professionals, these 'Notes' constitute a valuable record over time of changes in the condition of the patient. The evolution of each patient's situation is different, depending on the ailment and handicap involved. But the caregiver should note even changes or signs that may seem minor, but which a health professional may diagnose as significant. The caregiver can learn to observe the patient carefully in respect to some of the signs below. Some of these are obvious signs to note, but they are not exclusive; the observations to be recorded by the caregiver may be different from some of these, but no less revealing of an important development in the patient's health.

Movement

An overall reluctance to walk or lack of will to walk as far as usual.

Any sign of pain when the patient is walking or attempts to move. The specific location of the pain should be noted, along with any swelling or discoloration on the skin in the area of the pain.

- Stumbling or falling, even when there is no pain, or a fear of falling due to lack of balance.

- Warm or tender joints.

- Twitching or movements that are uncontrolled.

- Sensations of tingling or numbness in limbs or other parts of the body.

Nutrition

- Frequent thirst or lack of thirst.

- Changes in appreciation for favorite foods or sudden cravings for certain types of food.

- Change in the quantity of food taken, or in the timing for meals such as loss of appetite in the mornings or at noon.

- Weight loss.

- Refusal to take food.

- Pain before or after eating.

- Teeth or gum pains, evident when eating or drinking.

- Difficulty chewing or swallowing.

Mood and behavior

- Change in sleeping pattern, or patient wakes up at night and has difficulty returning to sleep, nightmares, tossing and turning.

- Unusual tiredness or drowsiness.

- Recurrent irritability, anger or withdrawal.

- Hallucinations.

- Obvious difficulty in remembering simple things, or confusion.

- Recurring anxiety.

- Depression.

- Emotional responses that are unusual for the patient.

Elimination

- Irregularity in bowel movements.

- Excreta of odd color, texture or amount.

- Faintness during bowel movements.

- Color, amount and odor of any vaginal discharge.

- Sores or pain in the area of the penis.

- Pain during bowel movements or when urinating.

- Frequent bowel movements or urination.

- Blood in the urine.

- Pain the area of the kidney.

Skin

- Skin rashes or persistent itching in specific areas of the body.

- Has a mole changed shape or become dark? Has a new one appeared, and where?

- Changes in color of lips, nails or extremities.

- Warm spots on, dryness or firmness of the skin.

- Bedsores.

Chest and abdomen

- Take note of any pain in the chest. If possible, ascertain its precise location and type of pain (sharp, stabbing, dull ache).

- Slow or accelerated pulse.

- Note any lumps, discharge or soreness in breasts.

- Bouts of wheezing or shortness of breath.

- Persistent cough.

- Changes in the color or consistency of saliva or mucus.

- Note stomach pain along with location and type of pain.

Take note of vomiting, the conditions prior to and after vomiting. Note any pain or nausea associated with vomiting.

Head

Frequency and intensity of headaches, along with type of pain and location.

Discharge or pain from the ears, or notable loss of hearing.

Pain in the eyes, blurring of vision, discharge or redness, and sensitivity to light.

Sores around the lips and inside the mouth.

Pain in the nasal area, and bleeding or discharges from the nose.

General

Temperature.

Pulse.

Blood pressure

Medications

Any change in response to medications,

New side effects after the taking of medication. Note the type of response – nausea, drowsiness, etc.

How to communicate observations to a physician or nurse ● ● ●

The observations written down in the caregiver's 'Notes' should all be communicated to the health professional. The caregiver should not feel this is an imposition. The presence of the physician or nurse is an opportunity to review the patient's condition and, if necessary, to make revisions in the program of treatment. The physician or nurse will appreciate the caregiver's observations. But, the time they have to devote to the patient is necessarily limited. Recognizing this, the caregiver will be as brief, descriptive and thorough as possible in reporting the observations and in answering specific questions by the physician or nurse about any of these.

When to call for help

Caregivers tend to develop a sense of pride in their own ability to provide for their patient. This sometimes makes them reluctant to concede the onset of a crisis. Realizing this is important, because it enables the caregiver to be rational about knowing when to call for help. Any situation that is abnormal, in which the patient is in obvious distress and the caregiver does not know what to do is a cause for getting assistance, using the relevant emergency numbers included in the caregiver's care plan. A copy of these emergency numbers should be positioned close to any fixed telephone or posted in an obvious location for use by anyone with a mobile telephone. Better yet, the caregiver can resort to a crisis plan that has been prepared in advance, in consultation with relevant specialists, as explained below.

The patient should be kept calm and as comfortable as possible while help is on the way.

Planning for a crisis

All the lessons a caregiver needs to learn about being prepared, informed and able to be an advocate for the patient come into play when a crisis occurs. The very nature of such an event is to be unexpected, although an attentive caregiver will know when a crisis is more likely to happen than not. The plan to deal with the crisis should assume it will be a surprise – for the caregiver, for the patient and for everyone able to come to their assistance. That is why common sense applied well in advance of a crisis comes to the rescue when it befalls. The organized caregiver will already have prepared a list of individuals or services to alert in the event of a crisis, with telephone numbers, names and any other relevant information (e.g. the name and number of a substitute if the regular physician is unavailable). Any medication prescribed for use in an emergency should be available, along with any special equipment that may have been prescribed. Such equipment should be cleaned and tested occasionally to ensure it will function properly when needed in an emergency situation.

A list of tasks to carry out in the event of a crisis should be kept in a place that is accessible to anyone who may have to deal with the emergency, since it can occur when the caregiver is absent or being replaced by someone else.

The plan should anticipate as much as possible the type of crisis to be dealt with, as the corresponding actions may be different from one cause of crisis to another. Figure 8.1 shows what a written crisis plan could look like.

Problem list	Intervention strategy/referrals
Fall	
Reaction to medication	
Difficulty breathing	
Unconsciousness	

Figure 8.1

An example of a crisis plan

The problem list will vary depending on the condition of the patient. The caregiver needs to consult a physician, nurse and/or other relevant specialist in advance, while preparing the plan, to determine the best strategy for dealing with the probable causes of a crisis. This will also help determine in which order to carry out the tasks to deal with the crisis, including whom to call or what service to alert.

How to communicate during a crisis • • •

When your patient is experiencing a medical crisis, the ability to observe symptoms carefully and report them accurately can be, literally, life-saving. But a crisis is also a time when it may be difficult for a caregiver to function clearly. With this in mind, it is important to anticipate moments of crisis, with the preparation of a checklist to be followed, for observations to be noted, and for actions to be taken. Keep the crisis action plan in a binder with the care plan. It should be reviewed along with the care plan by anyone replacing the caregiver. The list should include:

- The exact time the problem began.

- Any special circumstances observed when the problem began.

- Any thoughts or suggestions about what might have caused the problem.

- The first symptom noticed.

- Other symptoms that were observed.

- Any comments made by the patient when the problem began.

- Whether the symptoms came on abruptly or gradually.

- If the patient was receiving any medication or treatment just before the problem started. If so, what the medication or treatment was.

- Whether the patient made any comment after the problem started and as it progressed and, if so, what it was.

- Whether the patient has a history of this kind of problem. If so, the timing of the previous occasion and the diagnosis at that time.

- Any measures taken by the caregiver to assist the patient prior to the arrival of a health professional.

- Any measure that seemed to have a positive or negative effect.

The patient who has fallen

A fall is always cause for alarm, for both the patient and the caregiver. However, the latter needs to remain calm and analytical, while also moving expeditiously to deal with the fall. Once on the ground, the patient is safe for the moment and the situation must be assessed. It may be necessary to make the patient comfortable until help arrives. The patient should be assessed for possible injuries before this is done, or before any movement is attempted. The patient may be found to be uninjured and able to stand up, with or without assistance. If there is any doubt, help should be sought immediately.

Falls risk assessment

Falls can be the result of purely accidental circumstances, such as tripping. But it is possible to assess in advance the risk of a harmful fall occurring. A physician or nurse can help the caregiver with a falls risk assessment, to evaluate the risk that a patient will experience a fall. Various tools exist to carry out such an assessment, based on the patient's condition, medications being taken, and the patient's mental and emotional status. Where the risk is considerable the medical specialist can advise on measures that can be taken to reduce the risk, including the use of any special equipment such as canes or walking stands.

Caring for the Carer

Notes on Nursing – Florence Nightingale

The focus of the advice in *Notes on Nursing* is the patient. But Florence Nightingale experienced in her own life the wear and stress that can befall a caregiver. Although never one to spare herself or the caregivers she was seeking to inspire, she nonetheless included in her 'Notes' the message that caregivers should also care for themselves, by accepting that their unending presence at the side of their patient took a toll from which both could suffer. She insisted that the caregiver must understand that planning to be replaced at regular periods, and doing it so that someone else had everything at hand to offer the care that was needed, was also one of the important responsibilities to be assumed by a caregiver.

Caring for the carer today

The role of the caregiver is not a new phenomenon. It was an important element of care for the ill and injured in Florence Nightingale's time and it remains a key element in every country's strategy to deal with an increasing number of patients requiring care.

Caregivers around the world care for individuals from all age groups, across all stages of life, and across the continuum of care. Their needs, networks, resources, strengths and limitations vary from caregiver to caregiver and from one region or country to another. What unites them in their role is a concern for and a commitment to those in their care. However, the role also brings with it, in varying degrees, a set of risks and hazards that can befall anyone assuming this difficult role.

In developed countries, the aging of the population means that more individuals become candidates for care at home, rather than in institutions, for at least part of their old age. It also means that many of the caregivers are old themselves. A Canadian study of caregivers presents a picture that is typical for developed countries. It found, for example, that:

- Caregivers are predominantly female (77%) and typically older than the population at large, with 70% of them over 45 years old.

- The majority of people who receive care are aged between 75 and 85 years.

- Caregivers are most likely to report that they provide care out of a sense of family responsibility (67%).

- 52% of caregivers believe they had a choice about taking on their caregiving responsibilities.

- 50% of caregivers report health problems due to caregiving, with 79% of them admitting emotional difficulties due to caregiving.

- Almost seven in ten caregivers report that they need a break from their caregiving responsibilities, either frequently (21%) or occasionally (47%).

- The most significant predictor of caregiver 'stress' is the lack of choice about taking on the caregiving responsibilities.

- The majority of caregivers derive psychological benefits from providing care, including a sense of being able to make a positive contribution to the welfare of the care receiver (79%), and experiencing a strengthening of a valued relationship (90.6%).

In many countries, caregivers can often rely on outside services for support in providing care. However, in some countries the situation for caregivers is often not as good, with many having to earn a hard living for their family while at the same time providing care, often to more than one patient. In sub-Saharan Africa, women are traditionally considered the caregivers in the families if a family member falls sick. Family caregiving occurs under extremely limited conditions within the home, and there is very limited access to the formal healthcare system. With the dramatic spread of HIV/AIDS, family caregiving has reached new levels.

In many of the hardest-hit nations, women and girls take on the major share of providing care, often while also assuming responsibility for the children of the ill, or for the growing numbers of orphans. In these countries, the work of providing care is often done while continuing to work for an income or cultivate crops, which are often their family's only means of support.

Caring for an AIDS patient is difficult in any country. In a poor country it can be disastrous. One study found that, a woman in a rural community in Southern Africa must collect 24 buckets of water a day, by hand, and sometimes over a considerable distance, to care for a family member who is dying of AIDS – water to wash the clothes, the sheets and the patient after regular bouts of diarrhea. In many countries, the care provided by a family member at home is the only option available. It is estimated that up to 90% of care due to illness in the region is home-based. According to UNAIDS, two-thirds of primary caregivers in households surveyed in Southern Africa are female; one-quarter of these are over 60 years of age. A South African national evaluation of home-based care found that 91% of caregivers were women.

The difficulties of caring and giving care ● ● ●

Providing care on a regular basis for a cherished relative or other individual is physically tiring; it can also be a drain on the emotions and a source of anxiety, which can lead to feelings of inadequacy or resentment. Even the best good-will combined with a generous spirit can succumb to the unrelenting needs of a patient whose suffering and discomfort are shared every day by the caregiver.

It is frequent for caregivers to assume an attitude of self-abnegation, where they will deny their own feelings of inadequacy or resentment. Caregivers often assume their role out of necessity, because there is no one else to do it properly, but there is also a certain degree of altruism arising from their sense of responsibility in human relationships and families. This leaves caregivers vulnerable to the repression of emotions and physical symptoms that run counter to their image of what it means to be an ideal caregiver. This behavior needs to be recognized by every caregiver as a typical response to a difficult situation; every caregiver will experience some variation of this 'normal' condition. But, caregivers need also to realize that their own physical and mental well-being cannot be put into jeopardy in the process of providing care; both the caregiver and the patient will suffer from ignoring this basic reality. To help prevent falling into a situation of burnout, it is essential that caregivers take time for themselves. The relentless suffering or discomfort of a patient is often a goad to do too much, assume too much, and take on more of the burden than one person can stand.

A patient can be as demanding as the ailment or circumstances that he or she must live with. To deal with insistent demands requires calm, and recourse to the care plan, with adjustments if necessary. It is important to separate the patient from the ailment or condition, and to avoid blaming the patient for the situation in which both the patient and the caregiver must live. This is why every caregiver must include in the overall care plan provision for enough time and energy to account for their own physical and mental well-being. This is not a luxury, but an absolute requirement for anyone who anticipates providing care over a significant period of time.

The caregiver's first responsibility should be to ensure that he or she is able to sustain the effort to provide personal care for the patient. Above all, this means a responsibility to keep oneself healthy, balanced and strong. This can include:

- Eating a healthy diet rich in fruits, vegetables and whole grains and low in saturated fat.

- Trying to get enough sleep and rest.

- Finding time for exercise. Regular exercise can help reduce stress and improve health in many ways.

- Seeing a healthcare provider for a check-up, including discussion of any symptoms of depression or illness.

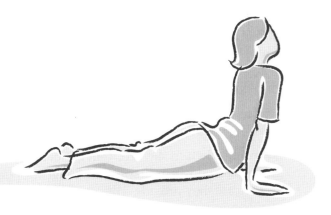

Figure 9.1

Exercise is beneficial to health in many ways and can reduce the stress of caring for a loved one

- Staying in touch with friends. Social activities can help keep a feeling of being connected and help with stress.

- Maintaining interests, such as reading, sports, community activities, etc.

- Reserving a reasonable amount of time for enjoyable pursuits and hobbies, such as sports, gardening or having a regular massage.

- Ensuring that there are people available who can provide respite in providing care, and that they are provided with everything they need. A well-prepared care plan that is easy to consult and follow will greatly reduce the caregiver's inevitable worry or guilt about being absent.

- Consulting health professionals about any concerns involving health and morale. This is not a luxury, but a reasonable precaution.

- Accepting the luxury of feeling tired, frustrated or angry, while accepting always that these are normal, human emotions that are natural under the circumstances faced by a caregiver. The caregiver needs to find a means of getting rid of guilt, anger and frustration in whatever way works best for them; this can be through physical activity, socializing with friends, or keeping a written account or diary of their time spent as a caregiver.

- Accepting personal limitations, and coping with these by seeking advice or assistance.

- Knowing when to say 'No'. Caregivers need to set limits beyond which they can no longer be effective in the care they provide. This can be in terms of the demands from others, or demands from a patient that go beyond the care needed, or which cannot be fulfilled without putting the caregiver's well-being at risk.

- Understanding that caregiving is a unique role, different from that of being a spouse or a relative, which calls on the development of skills and the exercise of different talents.

- Speaking up. Most caregivers tend not to recognize that they fulfil a special role in society – seeing the work they do simply as a manifestation of their concern and affection. This makes them reluctant to speak up about their likes, dislikes and needs, fearing that such remarks will be taken as complaining.

- Learning to say 'Yes' to offers of help. Have a list ready when someone offers to lend a hand, whether it's grocery shopping or staying with a loved one. This not only helps the caregiver, but gives others the satisfaction that they are providing support for the person giving care.

- Creating a support network. Caregivers often feel they carry their burden alone. However, most have friends, family, church groups or other support groups who are ready and willing to lend a hand. Use this available support to maintain your health and relieve stress.

- A caregiver must take care of their own health, and must not ignore medical appointments or examinations.

- Taking a break, by making a schedule that provides time off for other activities. A plan should be made with other family members, friends or home health aides to provide respite for the caregiver on a regular basis.

The health of the caregiver: how to manage physical strain and stress • • •

Providing care for a loved one is rewarding, but it can also lead to damaging levels of stress. Studies of caregivers often identify stress and the risk it represents for the caregiver's health as the primary issue to be addressed. The stress felt by caregivers is often unique in that it is typically an ongoing, long-term, 'chronic' condition, frequently made worse by the fact that the patient is someone for whom the caregiver feels strong bonds of love or affection. Such sustained stress, made worse by feelings of resentment combined with guilt, can help provoke health risks such as high blood pressure, heart conditions, arthritic flare-ups, acid reflux, head, neck and back aches, and other serious conditions. Stress can also lead to depression, which in time exacerbates health problems.

Because caregiving can be an all-consuming activity, monopolizing not only the caregiver's energy and time, but also their emotions, it can lead to disregard for healthy ways of living. Caregivers can fall into habits that are detrimental to themselves, ignoring signs about their own health and even disregarding the need for regular medical consultations. It is not unusual for caregivers to seek comfort from alcohol or prescription drugs, as a balm for their discomfort. Many cease exercising regularly or eating well. The cycle that is set up by an increased focus on providing care, leading to less attention to one's own needs, is ultimately destructive. The important message for caregivers is that their 'job' must include caring for themselves.

Depression

During a long convalescence or period of treatment, a caregiver will experience guilt about not being able to do enough or not being able to do it better. The onset of depression, which can become deleterious to the caregiver's own health and to the quality of care they can provide for the patient, presents a number of common symptoms.

- Persistent sadness and hopelessness.
- Sense of guilt and low self-worth.

- Loss of interest in your own life and pleasures, friends, hobbies and sports.

- Fatigue and tiredness.

- Lack of concentration and poor memory.

- Insomnia, bad dreams.

- Changes in appetite and weight.

- Dire thoughts about death and living.

- Lack of patience, and irritability.

- Anger and resentment.

A combination of such symptoms has to be taken seriously and needs to be discussed with a health specialist.

Effective communication ● ● ●

Being able to communicate constructively is one of a caregiver's most important tools. By communicating in ways that are clear, assertive and constructive, a caregiver will maintain a better relationship with the person being cared for, and with other individuals involved in providing care. Good communication is an individual talent, but there are some simple rules that can help anyone in communicating with someone in their care.

- *Use 'I' messages rather than 'you' messages*. Saying 'I feel angry' rather than 'You made me angry' enables you to express your feelings without placing the blame on someone else, or causing them to become defensive. This approach enables you to assume responsibility for your feelings and reactions, but it also places the onus on the patient to recognize some responsibility in provoking them.

- *Respect the rights and feelings of others*. The hours spent with a patient provide the caregiver with an unusual, intimate knowledge of the person. It also builds a level of trust that needs to be maintained.

A patient has a right to privacy, which the caregiver must respect. The caregiver learns about the patient's foibles and aspects of life about which the patient may feel protective or defensive. A caregiver must never use any of this information intentionally to hurt the person's feelings, but also needs to be clear about being treated with the same respect.

- *Empathy.* Often, empathy is required to accept that a person in pain or discomfort will sometimes react with resentment or with words that are injurious or upsetting. When this is unusual it needs to be accepted as such, if it becomes a pattern it needs to be discussed openly.

- *Be clear and specific.* Speak directly to the patient. Don't hint or hope that the patient will guess what is meant or what is being asked. When a caregiver speaks directly about needs and feelings, there is always a risk that the patient might disagree or say no to a request. A caregiver should be prepared to accept that the patient has a right to personal opinions and that the fact of giving care does not oblige a patient to accept every opinion or request. When both parties speak openly and directly, the chances of reaching an understanding are much greater; the relationship can only benefit from being aware of each other's ideas and opinions, especially those where an honest difference is recognized and accepted for what it is.

- *Be a good listener.* It is often said, but worth repeating, that listening is the most important aspect of communication. If anything being said is not clear, it is better to inquire than to surmise.

Respite care ● ● ●

The term 'respite care' usually refers to an extended period of 'time off' for a caregiver during which the patient's care is assumed by someone else, either at home or in an institution. The replacement caregiver may be a health professional, a family member or a friend of the patient.

The caregiver who experiences the need for such an extended break should discuss it with a health professional, to review the circumstances and the options available. It is normal for someone who has assumed responsibility for the care of a loved one to feel guilt and reluctance about such a course. In many cases, however, it can be beneficial to both the patient and the caregiver. Once again, this should be discussed openly with a health professional, who can draw on their experience to provide advice.

Respite care does not work wonders for everyone involved in all cases. Many caregivers simply 'miss' their loved one during an extended leave, or experience an increase in stress that offsets any possible advantage of an extended leave. The decision to have recourse to respite care needs to be considered carefully in all respects, including the health of the caregiver and the effects on the patient.

The type and duration of respite care should also be discussed with all concerned.

The anxiety felt by most caregivers during respite care is usually rooted in concerns for the well-being of the patient. These can be relieved to some extent by making available to those who will provide respite care the detailed care plan that the caregiver has developed and kept up to date.

Caring for a patient who is terminally ill ● ● ●

The difficulty of being constantly present as a loved one slips into death is a reality for caregivers. As with all aspects of providing care, the challenges and emotional difficulties encountered can best be dealt with by anticipation and planning. When there is no possibility of recovery, and death is inevitable, the caregiver can still do a great deal to help the patient die peacefully and with dignity.

At some point the patient may not be able to make decisions about medical treatment. At this time such decisions are given over to a close family member, who may be the caregiver, and to the patient's physician. In many countries it is possible for an individual to prepare an advance directive to cover such an eventuality. This is usually a legal document, which can include a power of attorney or what is known as a 'living will.' Such a document may include a general statement about the patient's preferences concerning life-saving measures and medical treatment. Some advance directives contain lists of specific medical treatments that the patient does or does not wish to receive. Such documents need to be prepared well in advance of their being needed. Family and friends should be informed well in advance of their existence, preferably by the patient.

(A living will is a legal document with written instructions for health professionals and loved ones about the patient's wishes in terms of treatment to be applied after the patient is no longer able to make such decisions. The legal status of living wills varies from one jurisdiction to another, and it is best to consult a legal professional about legal provisions applying in any specific situation.)

In some cases the patient may need to be moved from home care to an institution. This decision is usually taken by family members in consultation with health professionals. However, if the last days of the patient's life are to be lived at home, there is a great deal the caregiver can do to provide comfort. There are conditions that arise in most cases of terminal illness that can be anticipated and alleviated in consultation with health professionals. Their experience will be useful in anticipating problems that may arise for a specific patient, and how these can be dealt with, perhaps through the use of special techniques, equipment or medication. Some of these conditions include:

- Constipation is common for many terminal illnesses.
- Drinking and eating problems.
- Difficulty breathing.

- Vomiting and nausea.
- Frequent hiccups (involuntary contractions of the diaphragm).
- Itching.
- Pain.

The control of pain may be the single most useful function of the physician and the caregiver in the final phase of a terminal illness. The physician will prescribe pain-killing medication appropriate to each circumstance, and it will often be up to the caregiver to ensure that this is given as and when it should be. Caregivers need to pay continuing attention to the side effects of the medications being used, and to discuss these with a health professional.

Health professionals may also recommend other methods for relief of pain, including relaxation techniques such as deep breathing, meditation and massage. The sooner a patient learns to use such methods, the more likely they are to be effective.

It is common for someone who is dying to experience moments of anxiety and agitation, sometimes manifested as insomnia, restlessness or groaning. Such behavior should be discussed with a health professional, who can determine if there is a medical solution, such as anti-anxiety medication.

In some cases the anxiety may be caused by unresolved personal issues that are disturbing the patient. The caregiver should discuss this with a health professional. In such cases it may be best to advise a close family member who can intervene with the patient. In some situations, the best course may be to call on the services of a member of the clergy, who can provide the patient with spiritual guidance.

The death of a patient ● ● ●

Death occurs as the body's systems shut down. This may have a sudden onset or take place gradually, depending on the patient's illness and condition. The health professionals providing treatment to the patient will be able to advise on the onset of death. Even in the final moments of life, we all crave contact with each other; during this time, the caregiver, family members and other loved ones can help by their presence and their attention, such as by holding the patient's hand and speaking of their affection. The signs that death has occurred include cessation of breathing and heartbeat, and a total lack of responsiveness. A health professional will make the final determination.

The arrangements for their funeral and interment can be anticipated well in advance of the patient's death. It will be a comfort to all concerned to know that the necessary arrangements have been discussed and agreed to, and that everything has been organized with the appropriate inter-venors (clergy, funeral services, etc.).

Grieving a loss

The experience of grief at the loss of a loved one is especially difficult for a caregiver, who has become accustomed to devoting time and energy to providing care. The emotions experienced are powerful, and can at times seem overwhelming. It is normal to give oneself time and space to grieve. But, as in all aspects of the role of a caregiver, the most damaging effects can be avoided by anticipation, planning and an awareness of the realities of grief. Each person experiences grief in an individual way, but grief tends to manifest itself through a process that is common to many people. The stages of grief that a caregiver can anticipate include:

- A profound sense of loss, felt as numbness or shock.

- A sense of denial, rooted in an unwillingness to accept the loss of a loved one.

- A gradual acceptance of the death and loss, accompanied by profound sadness and the release of feelings by weeping.

- A sense of guilt based on feeling that more could have been done by the caregiver and by others.

- Feelings of anxiety and a sense of disorganization, with the inability to concentrate and bouts of panic.

- Lingering feelings of loneliness and longing, accompanied by disinterest in the common activities of life, even those that were once a source of pleasure or relief.

- Intense feelings of anger or resentment, which may even be directed at the person who has died.

- The eventual acceptance of the patient's death, and a return to a life where their death remains a reality but not a dominant force.

Most of all, caregivers need the attention and care of other people in times of grief. This normal, human need should be anticipated. Caregivers can make sure they are surrounded by family and friends. Many communities also offer support through church or social groups for those who are grieving.

In some cases it may be wise for a caregiver to seek professional advice when experiencing grief that they feel they cannot handle by themselves. There are signs of needing help to which every caregiver should be attentive, including:

- Withdrawal from contact with family members and friends.

- Powerful feelings of hostility.

- Reliance on drugs or alcohol.

- Confused emotions, exuberance alternating with profound depression.

Becoming a victim to any of these possible consequences of grief can be avoided by anticipating the need to deal with the realities of grief, and planning to take the steps needed to overcome them.

10

Health Literacy for Caregivers

The work of a caregiver is usually based on generosity and bonds of affection. That is the caregiver's greatest strength, but it is not enough. Everyone in such a position needs to learn how to become an effective provider of care, so that the effort expended produces the best result for the patient, and for the caregiver. What we call 'health literacy' today, was also a preoccupation in Florence Nightingale's time.

Knowledge of the laws of health ● ● ●

As she notes in her Conclusion to *Notes on Nursing*, it is not the job of a caregiver to replace the physician or the nurse. Building a working relationship with these health professionals is, however, part of the caregiver's responsibility. Effective communications among such a team depends on the caregiver learning at least the basics about the patient's condition and how to provide the type and quality of care that will meet the patient's needs. Florence Nightingale called this 'knowledge of the laws of health' or 'sanitary knowledge'. Today, this apprenticeship in the basic rules of hygiene and of caregiving is part of what is generally referred to as health literacy. This chapter begins with Florence Nightingale's remarks on that and related subjects. It continues with guidance on health literacy for today's caregivers and patients. The Internet and other virtual or real networks are a component of what it means today for a caregiver to be 'literate' about health, and so the chapter concludes with guidance on sources of information and assistance available to the caregiver through these modern means of self-education.

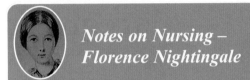

Notes on Nursing – Florence Nightingale

Nevertheless let no one think that because sanitary nursing is the subject of these notes, therefore, what may be called the handicraft of nursing is to be undervalued. A patient may be left to bleed to death in a sanitary palace. Another who cannot move himself may die of bed-sores, because the nurse does not know how to change and clean him, while he has every requisite of air, light, and quiet. But nursing, as a handicraft, has not been treated of here for three reasons:

That these notes do not pretend to be a manual for nursing, any more than for cooking for the sick; That the writer, who has herself seen more of what may be called surgical nursing, i.e. practical manual nursing, than, perhaps, any one in Europe, honestly believes that it is impossible to learn it from any book, and that it can only be thoroughly learnt in the wards of a hospital; and she also honestly believes that the perfection of surgical nursing may be seen practised by the old-fashioned "Sister" of a London hospital, as it can be seen nowhere else in Europe.

While thousands die of foul air, &c., who have this surgical nursing to perfection, the converse is comparatively rare.

Both for children and for adults, both for sick and for well (although more certainly in the case of sick children than in any others), I would here again repeat, the most frequent and most fatal cause of all is sleeping, for even a few hours, much more for weeks and months, in foul air, a condition which, more than any other condition, disturbs the respiratory process, and tends to produce "accidental" death in disease. I need hardly here repeat the warning against any confusion of ideas between cold and fresh air. You may chill a patient fatally without giving him fresh air at all. And you can quite well, nay, much better, give him fresh air without chilling him. This is the test of a good nurse. In cases of long recurring faintnesses from disease, for instance, especially disease which affects the organs of breathing, fresh air to the lungs, warmth to the surface, and often (as soon as the patient can swallow) hot drink, these are the right remedies and the only ones. Yet, oftener than not, you see the nurse or mother just reversing this; shutting up every cranny through which fresh air can enter, and leaving the body cold, or perhaps throwing a greater weight of clothes upon it, when already it is generating too little heat. "Breathing carefully, anxiously, as though respiration were a function which required all the attention for its performance," is cited as a not unusual state in children, and as one calling for care in all the things enumerated above. That breathing becomes an almost voluntary act, even in grown up patients who are very weak, must often have been remarked. "Disease having interfered with the perfect accomplishment of the respiratory function, some sudden demand for its complete exercise, issues in the sudden standstill of the whole machinery," is given as one process: – "life goes out for want of nervous power to keep the vital functions in activity," is given as another, by which "accidental" death is most often brought to pass in infancy. Also in middle age, both these processes may be seen ending in death, although generally not suddenly. And I have seen, even in middle age, the "sudden stand-still" here mentioned, and from the same causes. To sum up: the answer to two of the commonest objections urged, one by women themselves, the other by men, against the desirableness of sanitary knowledge for women, plus a caution, comprises the whole argument for the art of nursing.

Real knowledge of the laws of health alone can check this.

It is often said by men, that it is unwise to teach women anything about these laws of health, because they will take to physicking, – that there is a great deal too much of amateur physicking as it is, which is indeed true. One eminent physician told me that he had known more calomel given, both at a pinch and for a continuance, by mothers, governesses, and nurses, to children than he had ever heard of a physician prescribing in all his experience. Another says, that women's only idea in medicine is calomel and aperients. This is undeniably too often the case. There is nothing ever seen in any professional practice like the reckless physicking by amateur females.

But this is just what the really experienced and observing nurse does not do; she neither physics herself nor others. And to cultivate in things pertaining to health observation and experience in women who are mothers, governesses or nurses, is just the way to do away with amateur physicking, and if the doctors did but know it, to make the nurses obedient to them – helps to them instead of hindrances. Such education in women would indeed diminish the doctor's work, but no one really believes that doctors wish that there should be more illness, in order to have more work.

What pathology teaches. What observation alone teaches. What medicine does. What nature alone does.

It is often said by women, that they cannot know anything of the laws of health, or what to do to preserve their children's health, because they can know nothing of "Pathology," or cannot "dissect," – a confusion of ideas which it is hard to attempt to disentangle. Pathology teaches the harm that disease has done. But it teaches nothing more. We know nothing of the principle of health, the positive of which pathology is the negative, except from observation and experience. And nothing but observation and experience will teach us the ways to maintain or to bring back the state of health. It is often thought that medicine is the curative process. It is no such thing; medicine is the surgery of functions, as surgery proper is that of limbs and organs. Neither can do anything but remove obstructions; neither can cure; nature alone cures. Surgery removes the bullet out of the limb, which is an obstruction to cure, but nature heals the wound. So it is with medicine; the function of an organ becomes obstructed; medicine, so far as we know, assists nature to remove the obstruction, but does nothing more.

And what nursing has to do in either case, is to put the patient in the best condition for nature to act upon him. Generally, just the contrary is done. You think fresh air, and quiet and cleanliness extravagant, perhaps dangerous, luxuries, which should be given to the patient only when quite convenient, and medicine the *sine qua non*, the panacea. If I have succeeded in any measure in dispelling this illusion, and in showing what true nursing is, and what it is not, my object will have been answered.

Now for the caution.

It seems a commonly received idea among men and even among women themselves that it requires nothing but a disappointment in love, the want of an object, a general disgust, or incapacity for other things, to turn a woman into a good nurse. This reminds one of the parish where a stupid old man was set to be schoolmaster because he was "past keeping the pigs." Apply the above receipt for making a good nurse to making a good servant. And the receipt will be found to fail. Yet popular novelists of recent days have invented ladies disappointed in love or fresh out of the drawing-room turning into the war-hospitals to find their wounded lovers, and when found, forthwith abandoning their sick-ward for their lover, as might be expected. Yet in the estimation of the authors, these ladies were none the worse for that, but on the contrary were heroines of nursing. What cruel mistakes are sometimes made by benevolent men and women in matters of business about which they can know nothing and think they know a great deal.

The everyday management of a large ward, let alone of a hospital – the knowing what are the laws of life and death for men, and what the laws of health for wards – (and wards are healthy or unhealthy, mainly according to the knowledge or ignorance of the nurse) – are not these matters of sufficient importance and difficulty to require learning by experience and careful inquiry, just as much as any other art? They do not come by inspiration to the lady disappointed in love, nor to the poor workhouse drudge hard up for a livelihood.

And terrible is the injury which has followed to the sick from such wild notions! In this respect (and why is it so?), in Roman Catholic countries, both writers and workers are, in theory at least, far before ours. They would never think of such a beginning for a good working Superior or Sister of Charity. And many a Superior has refused to admit a Postulant who appeared to have no better "vocation" or reasons for offering herself than these.

It is true we make "no vows." But is a "vow" necessary to convince us that the true spirit for learning any art, most especially an art of charity, aright, is not a disgust to everything or something else? Do we really place the love of our kind (and of nursing, as one branch of it) so low as this? What would the Mere Angelique of Port Royal, what would our own Mrs. Fry have said to this?

I would earnestly ask my sisters to keep clear of both the jargons now current every where (for they are equally jargons); of the jargon, namely, about the "rights" of women, which urges women to do all that men do, including the medical and other professions, merely because men do it, and without regard to whether this is the best that women can do; and of the jargon which urges women to do nothing that men do, merely because they are women, and should be "recalled to a sense of their duty as women," and because "this is women's work," and "that is men's," and "these are things which women should not do," which is all assertion, and nothing more. Surely woman should bring the best she has, whatever that is, to the work of God's world, without attending to either of these cries. For what are they, both of them, the one just as much as the other, but listening to the "what people will say," to opinion, to the "voices from without?" And as a wise man has said, no one has ever done anything great or useful by listening to the voices from without.

You do not want the effect of your good things to be, "How wonderful for a woman!" nor would you be deterred from good things by hearing it said, "Yes, but she ought not to have done this, because it is not suitable for a woman." But you want to do the thing that is good, whether it is "suitable for a woman" or not. It does not make a thing good, that it is remarkable that a woman should have been able to do it. Neither does it make a thing bad, which would have been good had a man done it, that it has been done by a woman. Oh, leave these jargons, and go your way straight to God's work, in simplicity and singleness of heart.

Danger of physicking by amateurs.

I have known many ladies who, having once obtained a "blue pill" prescription from a physician, gave and took it as a common aperient two or three times a week – with what effect may be supposed. In one case I happened to be the person to inform the physician of it, who substituted for the prescription a comparatively harmless aperient pill. The lady came to me and complained that it "did not suit her half so well."

If women will take or give physic, by far the safest plan is to send for "the doctor" every time – for I have known ladies who both gave and took physic, who would not take the pains to learn the names of the commonest medicines, and confounded, e.g., colocynth with colchicum. This is playing with sharp-edged tools "with a vengeance."

There are excellent women who will write to London to their physician that there is much sickness in their neighbourhood in the country, and ask for some prescription from him, which they used to like themselves, and then give it to all their friends and to all their poorer neighbours who will take it. Now, instead of giving medicine, of which you cannot possibly know the exact and proper application, nor all its consequences, would it not be better if you were to persuade and help your poorer neighbours to remove the dung-hill from before the door, to put in a window which opens, or an Arnott's ventilator, or to cleanse and lime-wash the cottages? Of these things the benefits are sure. The benefits of the inexperienced administration of medicines are by no means so sure.

An almost universal error among women is the supposition that everybody must have the bowels opened once in every twenty-four hours, or must fly immediately to aperients. The reverse is the conclusion of experience. This is a doctor's subject, and I will not enter more into it; but will simply repeat, do not go on taking or giving to your children your abominable "courses of aperients," without calling in the doctor.

Health literacy

Whether in Florence Nightingale's time or now, it remains a fact that clear communication and the effective transfer of information are basic components required for quality healthcare. In a clinical setting, a healthcare provider must be able adequately to explain diagnoses, medical procedures and appropriate courses of action to a patient. Likewise, the patient should be able to describe symptoms, provide information on medical and social history and answer questions related to health conditions and well-being. The caregiver's role in this exchange of information falls somewhere in between, acting as an advocate for the patient, but also as an interpreter to facilitate the dialogue between health professionals and the patient. Besides this interpersonal communication, other sources, such as print brochures, DVDs and the Internet, provide information to patients about health behaviors, self-care, treatment decision-making, or directions for navigating a particular health system.

During this transfer of information, there is an assumption that the patient and the caregiver possess an adequate set of skills to understand the health messages provided to them and to take appropriate action in response. This may be challenging, as health information provided to patients frequently includes vague medical jargon and concepts that are unfamiliar to the average adult. While some patients may be able to comprehend health messages and act accordingly, others may not. Clear differences exist between patients in terms of cognitive ability and the level of activation needed to decode, process and derive meaning from oral or written information, and to engage in the necessary actions for appropriate care.

The concept of health literacy reflects a patient's ability to obtain and act upon health information, given the demands placed on the patient in an increasingly complex healthcare system. The generally accepted definition of health literacy is the 'degree to which individuals have the capacity to obtain, process, and understand basic health information and services needed to make appropriate health decisions'.

Health literacy is a multifaceted concept, of which reading ability is a fundamental component. While health literacy is intrinsically related to general literacy, it encompasses a broad range of cognitive and social processes beyond the ability to read, process and understand written materials.

Speaking and listening skills ● ● ●

Speaking and listening skills are essential, as individuals navigating a healthcare setting must be able to understand and engage in oral communication with healthcare providers in order to obtain and fully understand health information. Conceptual knowledge and numeracy skills, or the ability to perform basic arithmetic functions and apply mathematical knowledge to everyday tasks, are also important to an individual's ability to understand diagnoses, risks and the need for medical interventions.

As more demands are placed on patients and on caregivers by a complex healthcare system, more prerequisite skills are needed for them to have functional health literacy, or the ability successfully to navigate a healthcare system and interpret and act upon the health information given. Functional health literacy has become increasingly important as the gap widens between the average cognitive and social skills of adult health-seekers and the burdens placed on patients and families when attempting to access services in complex healthcare settings.

Health literacy and health outcomes ● ● ●

Over the past two decades, an increasing body of research has examined the relationship between limited health literacy and adverse health outcomes. Although the relationship is not entirely clear, there are plausible mechanisms by which health literacy could directly affect acquisition of health knowledge, health behaviors and compliance with medication and self-care regimens.

Over the past decade, few interventions have been formulated to address the problem of limited health literacy. While there is a need for additional research on how to respond appropriately to limited health literacy, certain health communication 'best practices' have been recommended by various professional medical organizations. These are relatively simple steps that will assist in identifying patients at risk due to limited health literacy and the associated potentially poor health outcomes, and will improve the quality and effectiveness of communication during clinical encounters.

It may not always be possible to identify patients with limited health literacy. A best practice for health communication is to adopt a universal precaution approach, and always to use plain language and to try to avoid the use of medical jargon. This is not always possible, so terms and concepts should be defined and clarified when they arise. Techniques for effective verbal communication are included in Table 10.1.

Limited health literacy is a serious barrier to communication in healthcare. Caregivers should ask that physicians, nurses and other medical professionals communicate with them and their patients in a clear and concise manner, and to provide easy to understand printed and visual materials to reinforce the health messages and instructions.

Sources of information for the caregiver   ● ● ●

Caregivers can be overwhelmed by the ongoing responsibilities of caring for a patient. They may recognize that they need additional help, but do not know how to ask or where to begin to find appropriate or affordable resources and support services in their communities. Although caregivers around the world may experience the same needs for support and information, they will not all be fortunate enough to have easy access to such services. Whatever their situation, caregivers will all benefit from knowing what types of services are available, and which of these will be of greatest use in their situation.

The most fortunate caregivers will have access to well-informed volunteers whose task it is to help them find support. These may be knowledgeable individuals in public institutions or members of voluntary community organizations. Where they exist, such volunteers can help caregivers

Table 10.1 Effective verbal communication techniques

Communication technique	Explanation
Talk slowly	Slow down the pace of speech when talking with a patient.
	An effective way to solicit questions would be to ask 'What questions do you have?' This is an open-ended question and allows the patient more room for possible interactive communication
Encourage questions	Questions such as 'Do you understand?,' 'Do you have questions?,' and 'Do you think you can (check your blood sugars now)?' are vague and give the patient the opportunity to avoid the question with a simple 'no' answer
Explain things in clear, plain language	Plain, non-medical language should be used. New terms should be defined. Words or expressions that are familiar to patients should be used, such as 'pain-killer' instead of 'analgesic'. Jargon, statistics, and technical phrases should be avoided
Avoid complex numeric concepts and statistics	Many people do not understand percentages. Patients do not understand all the numbers given to them before they make any treatment decision. Instead of saying, 'There is a 20% chance that you will experience outcome X', one can tell the patient '20 out of 100 people will experience outcome X'
Use analogies and metaphors	Analogies should be selected to relate complex concepts to things the patient already knows (e.g., "Arthritis is like a creaky hinge on a door")
Limit information provided	Limit information to 1–3 key messages per discussion. Reviewing and repeating each point helps reinforce the messages
Verify patient understanding	A "show me" method should be used to allow the patient to demonstrate understanding and for the caregiver to verify patient understanding
Avoid vague terms	Say "Take 1 hour before you eat breakfast" instead of "Take on an empty stomach"

to be assertive and proactive about seeking assistance; they can provide information about appropriate community services or organizations that might offer additional support. Volunteers will likely also be familiar with local organizations or Internet-based support groups designed to help caregivers, in some cases simply by giving them the opportunity to share their feelings and experiences. Many support groups are an excellent source of information on community resources, advice on care, and how to obtain assistance for specific situations.

When additional support is needed, it is important for caregivers to be able to act on these needs as quickly as possible. If specialized volunteers are not available, and in a situation where there are no community or institutional services, it is nonetheless important for the caregiver to seek whatever assistance is at hand. This will often be family members or friends and neighbors. There are moments when caregivers simply need to talk to someone about their experience of caregiving, and some of the difficulties they are dealing with. Caregivers need to recognize that this is a valid need, not a sign of flinching or irresponsibility, although those feelings will no doubt be present. Both the patient and the caregiver are at risk when such needs are ignored. Beyond the simple need to talk to someone, it is often a necessity for caregivers to look for other substantial forms of support.

This section has been prepared to help caregivers determine what kinds of support may be available to them and how to go about finding it. Not all the types of support described here are available in every community, but knowing what they are is a starting point in the process of identifying what is available, and in judging which of them can provide the kind of support required in specific situations. Armed with knowledge about support programs and organizations, references and other materials, caregivers can be more effective in finding information and services that may enhance the care they provide for their patients, the quality of their own caregiving experience and the quality of the life shared by both.

Where is the information? ● ● ●

Trying to obtain information about local services and resources to address the needs of a caregiver or patient can be challenging when one does not know where to look or the exact name of an organization or resource. Often, the best way to obtain local listings is to contact national or regional government organizations and institutions, particularly departments or agencies dealing with health and social issues. They will often have lists of organizations or even individuals who can provide different types of support. These sources can not only put people into contact with appropriate local affiliates or offices, they can also help explain the scope of services available at a particular community location.

Those in search of assistance can also contact local physicians, health clinics, special residences, a community pastor or a library to learn about support services that may be available. Libraries may be able to provide books and guides written for caregivers. Some of these groups may be able to supply a list of further contacts, depending on the needs of the caregiver. The organizations and agencies listed might be social organizations for men and women, or community-based business and social groups.

The types of support services that may be available in your community ● ● ●

An adult day services center is a local facility in which adults who cannot physically or mentally function on their own are provided with organized and well-supervised social activities and other support services. Adult day services centers often offer caregivers short-term respite care for valuable time off during the day. An adult day services center can also take care of the daily needs of a care recipient while the caregiver works during the day to earn a living. Adult day services centers provide benefits to care recipients through socialization activities and other services not available at home.

Local branches of organizations devoted to the support and care of those with particular conditions (e.g., Alzheimer's disease, multiple sclerosis) run adult day services programs that are designed to meet the special needs of those patients. If no local branch exists, the caregiver should enquire if there are regional or national groups, and if they can offer information or support.

Assistive devices ● ● ●

Assistive devices and aids for daily living are items and equipment designed to help incapacitated and disabled persons accomplish their activities of daily living more easily. These include: special products for the visually or hearing impaired; robotic devices designed to help with tasks; mechanical lifts to help people get in and out of bed or up and down stairs; walkers, hand rails and ramps to aid mobility; and incontinence and toileting products.

Information on assistive devices is available through companies that manufacture the devices and through non-profit organizations and agencies that provide information and services to individuals who have medical conditions that may warrant the need for assistive devices. Some of these companies and organizations offer additional services, such as insurance-claim processing and monthly product delivery – particularly useful for disposable products such as incontinence and ostomy products. Some national organizations dedicated to supporting patients with specific diseases or disabilities also offer equipment 'on loan.'

Caregiver support groups ● ● ●

Caregiver support groups allow caregivers to express their feelings, share skills and learn about caregiving issues in a supportive environment. Professionals and/or volunteers may lead such groups. If no such group is available in the caregiver's region, there may still be the option of accessing such groups on the Internet, through chatrooms, bulletin boards, websites and email exchanges. Some Internet support groups run 'topical' chatrooms on specific issues and situations, allowing participants to share information. Often, they will also include participation of professionals, from whom it is possible to obtain advice on dealing with specific situations.

Real or virtual support groups are also available for caregivers of patients with specific diseases, disorders or disabilities. Participating regularly in support groups can help caregivers develop relationships with others who are experiencing similar situations or feelings, and who can understand the challenges, stresses and fatigue associated with caring for a patient. Participating in support groups can also help alleviate the isolation that can be part of the caregiving experience.

Internet-based support has the advantage of letting caregivers reach out at their convenience, no matter what hour of the day or night. Access to a computer can be a problem, but most communities have Internet cafés, and schools and institutions may allow computer access for caregivers in special circumstances.

Legal advice ● ● ●

When a caregiver becomes responsible for managing the personal, medical and financial affairs of an older care recipient, legal issues often come into play. While the care recipient is lucid, the caregiver should obtain legal advice regarding how to set up a durable power of attorney, or help the care recipient create an advance medical directive or update a will. When a patient becomes cognitively impaired and unable to make decisions, the caregiver may need to obtain legal counsel about how to arrange for legal guardianship.

It is always a good idea to seek legal advice regarding how to address these situations. The patient may already have a professional relationship with a lawyer or law firm.

Other caregivers or caregiver organizations will sometimes be the best referrals to legal experts who are familiar with the situations that arise in providing care. Professional legal or medical associations, at local or regional level, can also be good sources of information for caregivers seeking legal advice.

Index

Note: Page numbers in *italics* refer to figures/illustrations.

dietary supplements, 59
disabilities, feeding tips for
    patients with, 78–9
disease, changing understanding
    of, 8–9
disease–drug interactions, 59–60
disinfectants, 17, 80–1
disinfection, food preparation
    surfaces/equipment, 80–1
drainage, 12
dressing
    helping patients, 120–2
    see also clothing
drugs see medicine/medication

E

eating aids, 82
effluvia, from excreta, 16
eggs, in diet, 74–5
elimination, 16–17, 100–2
    observations on, 137
emotions
    of caregivers, 148
    helping patient express, 122–3
    see also anxiety
equipment, medical, 22–3
exercise
    for carers, 147, 147
    for patients, 63
explanations to patient, 26–8

F

facial features, 132
faintness, 132–3
falling/falls, patient, 142
family members, xiii, 20–1, 145,
    149, 153–7, 171
fancies, patient, 34, 40
feeding
    aids, 82
    assistance for patient, 76–8
    rules, 71–3
    timing, and assistance, 72–3
    tips, 34, 76–9
    see also food
feelings, helping patient express,
    122–3

fever, 103, 104
fingernails, 107
first aid kit, 23–4
fitness, 63
flowers, 41
food
    appetite and, 129–31
    interactions with medicines,
        57–9
    leaving at bedside, 72
    nutritional observations, 136
    patient's diet, 73–5, 77, 130–1
    preparation, 81
    solid vs. liquid, 71–2, 131
    see also diet (patient's);
        feeding
fungal infections, 109–10
fungi, 103, 108–11

G

gloves, disposable, 107
good news, sharing, 117–18
gossiping, 119, 134
grab bars, 17, 21
grief management, 156–7
grooming, personal, 97–100, 99
guilt, 148, 150, 153, 157

H

handicaps, feeding tips for
    patients with, 78–9
handrails, 17, 21
hand-washing, 21–2, 22, 96–7,
    104–7, 106
    before food handling/meals,
        80–2
    infection prevention, 104–7
    method, 104–7, 106
head observations, 138
health
    caregiver's, 147, 147–9
    laws, 159–60, 161–2
    literacy, 166–7, 168–9
health insurance, 51, 67
health professionals/caregiver
    relationship, 50–3, 55–8,
    154–6, 167